More Praise For Mary MacCracken's

The Memory of All That

"A moving account of one couple's vibrant, loving relationship, their courage in facing Alzheimer's, and their fierce unwillingness to abandon any moment of shared happiness before the end. This poignant narrative also offers ways to handle the problems and difficult decisions faced by caregivers and their families."

—NANCY DUBLER, LLB, Affiliated Professor, Division of Medical Ethics, NYU Langone Medical Center and author of *Alzheimer's Dementia: Dilemmas in Clinical Research* and *Ethics on Call: A Medical Ethicist Shows How to Take Charge of Life-and-Death Choices*

"A road map for sustaining love in the face of inevitable loss for any of us. Mary MacCracken is a skilled storyteller who knows how to turn this tale of wrenching heartbreak into a surprisingly uplifting memoir."

—JAN MAHER, award-winning author of *The Persistence of Memory and Other Stories*, *Earth as It Is*, and *Heaven, Indiana*

"*The Memory of All That* is a generous and stirring memoir. MacCracken's gentle prose recounts her husband's decline into Alzheimer's and the toll it takes on them both. Her story, however, is not framed as tragedy but as a chronicle of married love—with no small share of laughter. Readers facing a similar journey will welcome this book with relief and hope"

—CHRISTINE HEMP, author of *Wild Ride Home: Love, Loss, and a Little White Horse*

"Mary MacCracken's book, *The Memory of All That*, is a love letter to her husband with dementia. Here but gone; no longer as he used to be. Ambiguous loss, it's called, with both "upwelling sadness" and "scraps of joy." In a world of loss right now, we can find solace in MacCracken's beautifully written story about love and purpose."

—PAULINE BOSS, PhD, author of *The Myth of Closure: Ambiguous Loss in a Time of Pandemic and Change* and *Loving Someone Who Has Dementia: How to Find Hope while Coping with Stress and Grief*

The
Memory
of
All That

The
Memory
of
All That

A Love Story About Alzheimer's

Mary MacCracken

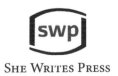

SHE WRITES PRESS

Published 2022

Printed in the United States of America

Print ISBN: 978-1-64742-417-6
E-ISBN: 978-1-64742-418-3
Library of Congress Control Number: 2022901591

For information, address:
She Writes Press
1569 Solano Ave #546
Berkeley, CA 94707

She Writes Press is a division of SparkPoint Studio, LLC.

For Cal MacCracken

May all know love like ours

Foreword

This beautifully told, heart-rending story describes Cal and Mary MacCracken's ordeal with Alzheimer's disease. More fundamentally, it is about how their deep, loving relationship remained central to their lives throughout and served as a potent tool in coping with the disease until the very end. As the book's subtitle indicates, this is truly a "love story." Mary reassures Cal soon after the appearance of some of the earliest cognitive signs of the disease that would gradually worsen and ultimately engulf him:

"We'll be okay. We have each other, and together we can handle anything."

Indeed they did handle "anything" and everything, despite formidable difficulties and immense suffering along the way.

Although there has been important progress in the field since Cal's illness in the 1990s, the disorder remains frustratingly elusive. There is still no cure, nor is there an effective method to prevent its appearance in the first place. We still do not have the ability to definitively diagnose Alzheimer's disease in a living person. Medication treatments currently available are only modestly helpful, at best, in slowing down the relentless progression of this disorder. But the crucial messages conveyed here so eloquently by Mary remain as important today as they were when Alzheimer's became a central feature of the Mac-Cracken's lives.

Both Cal and Mary MacCracken were excellent prob-lem-solvers. As a prolific, highly successful inventor, Cal had to manage the many difficulties along the path of transform-ing his ideas into successful creations. Mary, as well, needed to find effective methods of mastering the obstacles presented by the emotionally damaged and learning-disabled children with whom she worked. Cal and Mary enjoyed discussing their work together and no doubt learned a great deal from each other, not so much about energy storage or childhood disorders but about the importance of persevering, no matter how hopeless a situ-ation seemed, to find resolutions to whatever adversities arose.

In one sense, Alzheimer's can be viewed as an endless series of problems that confront the person with the illness and the caregiver. Mary was able to use her problem-solving skills, fueled by her great love for Cal, throughout the long ordeal of his illness. She became highly skilled at being able to helpfully respond to Cal's forgetfulness and myriad other symptoms. And she did so while striving to preserve Cal's pride and sense of self-worth, already damaged by the increasing struggles to function that he encountered as his illness took hold. This is always a major challenge for a caregiver of someone with Alz-heimer's disease or other form of dementia. It takes cleverness, a thorough understanding of the disease, and especially a deep-seated caring for the individual to be able to successfully balance these seemingly conflicting issues.

But no matter how resourceful and loving a caregiver may be, no one can manage Alzheimer's disease single-handedly. Although some caregivers feel that they should do just that, the effort to do so creates an overwhelming burden for the care-giver and is usually destined to fail. Mary was wise enough to turn to her family and close friends when she felt particularly overwhelmed, and was invariably comforted and reinvigorated by the support and understanding she received from them.

She also attended support groups for caregivers. It was vital to learn from others who were coping with similar challenges and who were able to empathize as only someone in a similar situation could. Attending a support group can be immensely helpful for anyone who has a loved one with the disease. Mary also found meeting individually with the social workers leading the support groups she attended, or others with experience with Alzheimer's, very useful. Yet too few caregivers take advantage of these critical aids, feeling that their challenges are "private," not to be shared with "strangers," or believing that they can somehow manage on their own. In most cases they can't.

Mary and Cal were fortunate to have the means to live at Kendal, a wonderful continuing care retirement community that has a very knowledgeable and compassionate staff and offers many comfortable and supportive amenities to those who reside there. No doubt, living at Kendal helped make this ordeal somewhat less terrible than otherwise. But it was their profound love for each other, Mary's commitment to and skill at solving problems, and her willingness to turn to family, friends, support groups, and others that were the crucial elements in helping Cal and Mary through this tragic saga. Anyone who has a loved one with Alzheimer's or another dementia should find valuable lessons and inspiration here.

—**Robert B. Santulli, MD,** author of
The Emotional Journey of the Alzheimer's Family and
The Alzheimer's Family: Helping Caregivers Cope

THEY CAN'T TAKE THAT AWAY
FROM ME

The way you wear your hat
The way you sip your tea
The memory of all that
No, they can't take that away from me

The way your smile just beams
The way you sing off key
The way you haunt my dreams
No, no, they can't take that away from me

We may never, never meet again,
on that bumpy road to love
Still I'll always, always keep the memory of
The way you hold your knife
The way we danced till three
The way you changed my life
No, no, they can't take that away from me

MUSIC AND LYRICS BY GEORGE GERSHWIN AND IRA GERSHWIN

Prologue

It was almost dark when I heard Cal's car pull into the driveway. I hurried down the stairs from my office, but Cal was already in the kitchen when I got there. He was standing very still, making no move to greet me.

"What?" I asked.

"Read this," he said quietly, holding out a letter.

"What is it?" Something was wrong. No hug. No kiss. Not like other nights.

"Just read it."

I skimmed the letter.

"We regret to inform you that we are unable to accept your application for long-term life insurance because of your existing condition of Alzheimer's disease."

"What's this about Alzheimer's disease? And when did you apply for long-term insurance?"

Cal shrugged. "Thought it was a good idea."

"And what about Alzheimer's?"

Another shrug.

This wasn't like Cal. We usually told each other everything—at least I thought we did. I certainly couldn't begin to guess what he was thinking now.

The Memory of All That

I rushed back up to my office over our garage, where I worked one-on-one with children and had just finished with a second grader struggling to read. Cal followed me, watching as I typed "Alzheimer's" into my computer.

Out loud I read to Cal, "Alzheimer's disease is a degenerative brain disorder that develops in mid-to-late adult life and results in a progressive"—I cleared my throat and skipped over the next two words, "and irreversible"—"decline in memory and various cognitive functions."

I stopped there and walked over to where Cal was standing and put my arms around him. "There must be some mistake. It was just last month that we went in to see that neurologist, that doctor who was so highly recommended. Neither of us liked him much. But even if we didn't, we did like what he told us: 'Just a mild memory loss, nothing serious.'"

Cal unwrapped my arms and led me to a chair. "Well, that's not what he told the insurance company. Here." He bent over the computer. "Let me read the rest of that."

I studied my handsome husband as he read. Jet-black hair, wide-set hazel eyes, ears close to his head, nose a little too long, slim athletic body. He was reading out loud clearly. It was true he had recently complained that he was having trouble spelling some words like "machine" and "consequences," but so did many of the other engineers in his office.

Cal shut down the computer and came over to rest his hand on my shoulder. "Well, thank you for finding that. At least we have some idea of what we're dealing with, and some of it makes sense. I tell you what though, if it turns out I do have Alzheimer's, you and I will beat it. And then we'll write a book about how we did it. Okay?"

"Okay," I answered, thinking how nothing ever really got Cal down. He just kept working away doggedly until he won.

I'd watched him come back in dozens of squash matches where he'd be behind five or more points, and then steadily, determinedly he'd fight back, winning point after point, until in the end he won the match. Nobody ever dared to count Cal out.

Even more impressive, before we married (a second marriage for us both) he'd had a calamitous misfortune with one of his inventions and had to declare bankruptcy. But he had paid off all his debtors, and now his company was successful, respected, and making money. Encouraged by him, I'd come back from losing my teaching job to setting up my own practice, and the books I'd written about the children I worked with had, after many rejections, been published. We were doing fine financially and were very much in love. It seemed nothing could stop us.

That night, lying in bed waiting for sleep to come, I smiled, remembering a time just before our wedding in June of 1969. We met at a favorite place, the Cloisters. We sat on the cliff in front of the massive building above the Hudson River and almost immediately Cal handed me a small box. He said, "A present for you."

I opened it and took out a silver bracelet with three charms. I touched each one. First a mask of joy and sorrow.

"We've known both," Cal said.

Then, a silver heart.

"Mine," he added.

I puzzled over the third charm and finally asked, "Cal, why did you give me a cash register?"

"Oh Lord," he said, taking the bracelet and studying the charm. "I thought it was a typewriter."

We laughed over this many times afterward and decided it was a lucky omen.

The Memory of All That

I rolled back into the hollow in the middle of our big bed and fitted myself against Cal's warm, sleeping body.

How could he have a degenerative, irreversible brain disease? It didn't seem possible.

Part I

BEFORE
ALZHEIMER'S

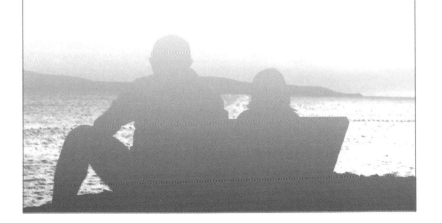

Chapter One

The first time I saw Cal, we didn't even speak. The second time, we chatted briefly at a party. The third time, when we were dancing together, he pushed me a little away. I glanced up at him questioningly and tried to move nearer, but he said, "Look at me; I want you to remember this."

"What?"

"I'm going to marry you someday."

I laughed. "How do you plan to do that? We're both already married, and we both have children we care about. Four for you, three for me."

Cal pulled me back in close to him and said, "Just remember what I told you."

I met Cal's father before I ever met Cal.

I had been married for eight years. My husband and I had three small children, a girl, Susan, age five, and twins, a boy and girl, Steve and Nan, age three. Stuart, my husband, worked for a large sales company and had been suddenly transferred to Poughkeepsie, New York.

We found an old Victorian house that we could rent. It had been modernized by its owners and had a brand-new kitchen. The downstairs walls, though, were painted an interesting lavender, and the living room was furnished with butterfly chairs and mobiles, a new decor for us. But the owners were very nice. The man of the house had been recalled to the Navy, and he and his wife were on their way to Washington, DC, for at least a year.

A few weeks before we were to move in, they graciously planned a party to introduce us to some of their friends. Dr. MacCracken, former president of Vassar College, was one of them. We were asked to come early, and Dr. MacCracken arrived shortly after we did. I was standing by the fireplace in the living room when he came over to me. He was a charming man and immediately engaged me in a conversation about college, going on to tell me about how important he thought education was for women. I was vaguely aware of other people arriving, but not until our hostess came and whispered, "I invited you to meet all my friends, not just one," did I realize how long we had been talking. I excused myself, but before I could leave, Dr. MacCracken stopped me and asked, "Where are you moving from and when?"

"From Tenafly, New Jersey, in about two weeks."

"Oh, that's too bad," he replied. "My son moved to Tenafly recently. You would have liked my son."

I forgot all about my conversation with Dr. MacCracken until some years later when I saw his son Cal for the first time on the paddle tennis courts in Englewood, New Jersey. Now I treasure his statement. It seems almost like a blessing.

Stuart and I lived in Poughkeepsie for two years. I had married him in June of 1945 when he was in the Navy. I had just turned nineteen and he was twenty-one. We were both too young to be married, but World War II was on, and he was about to ship out. Ten years later, he was out of the Navy, into sales, and no longer in love with me.

Mary MacCracken

In the spring of 1955, an uncle of his asked him to join the family firm, a large real estate operation based in Englewood, New Jersey, the town next to Tenafly. Stu was torn. He was heavily involved with another woman and had already told me that he no longer loved me, that there was someone else. But then the woman turned him down, and he decided to take his uncle up on the offer of a partnership.

I wanted to leave the marriage. I couldn't stand the thought of Stu touching me. But when I talked to my father to see if he could help me start a new life, he said he really couldn't. My mother was ill, and since my father had just retired, their funds were limited. He matter-of-factly pointed out that my options were few. I had no saleable skills, not even a college degree, since I'd left Wellesley after my sophomore year to marry Stu before he went overseas. Also, now, a decade later, I had three small children to care for and support. He advised that I put the past behind me and make a fresh start with our move back to Tenafly.

So, in the summer of 1955, we returned to the town where we had both gone to high school. We packed up our things, our strained marriage, and our children and moved back to what I thought of as home. We bought a house near the school that I had gone to as a little girl and registered my oldest daughter for second grade, and the twins for kindergarten. Although our marriage remained in a painful place, we were both trying to make our family work, and it was good to be back among old friends. We were all busy raising our children and working hard. Still, there was time for parties, friendly talk, and laughter. We joined an athletic club, and friends taught us a new game, paddle tennis.

That was where I first saw Cal. Stu and I were playing paddle tennis with friends on a cold, snowy Sunday when a man stopped to watch us. He was wearing a London Fog raincoat over tennis whites, and an old, slightly ridiculous gray fedora hat. But there was something about him . . .

"Who was that?" I asked my partner. "And how could he play tennis in this weather?"

"Not tennis. Squash. He's the club champion. In fact, he's won lots of squash awards. He's also the president of our club. His name is Calvin MacCracken. We call him Cal."

Cal lingered by the steps to the court. He was a stranger to me, but he looked so lonely. A big squash champ? Club president? How could he be lonely? I repeated his name under my breath, and from five years before, his father's words came back to me: "You would have liked my son."

Chapter Two

The Christmas holidays of 1958 were filled with festive parties and celebrations. Trees glittered on snow covered lawns, wreaths adorned front doors, and inside were more trees, poinsettias, and mistletoe. Fires and candles burned brightly. I remember standing at one buffet table, making a small turkey sandwich while music and laughter reverberated around me, thinking what fun it was to be back among the old crowd I'd grown up with and that maybe, maybe I could make my marriage work. Then someone spoke from behind me.

"I hear you've moved back from Poughkeepsie. I grew up there."

I turned, and there was Cal MacCracken smiling down at me.

From having seen Cal only twice in three years, I then seemed to see him everyplace. Our youngest daughters were in the same class at school, and since I was their room mother, I often ran into him there.

My husband was a good athlete and loved playing paddle tennis, as did Cal, so we were often around each other. We sometimes traveled together on fall and winter weekends when the two men played other clubs. The more Cal and I knew each other, the more we wanted to be together, and I guess we thought we could do it by just being friends. Of course, we couldn't. I think we began to realize that we should stay apart. But at the same time, we were inexplicably drawn together.

I had begun to work with autistic children and Cal was interested in the progress they were making, and I was fascinated by his inventing. How did he do it? How did his mind work?

I came to learn a lot about Cal in our talks. He'd gone to Princeton when only sixteen and majored in astronomy. But he'd always wanted to be an inventor and worked one summer with Thomas Edison's son, Theodore, in his lab in New Jersey. "If you want to do all the things you say you do," Theodore told Cal, "you'd better get an engineering degree." So, in 1940, the fall after graduating, Cal climbed in his old jalopy and drove to MIT.

A year later, in 1941, Cal had a degree in mechanical engineering and a job with General Electric in Schenectady, New York. The war was on. Britain, fighting hard to defend its shores, turned a secret project they had started, an early version of the jet engine, over to the US Department of Defense. The Department of Defense passed the project on to General Electric, which then gave it to a team of men known as the "hush-hush boys." Cal was assigned the task of designing a better combustion chamber for the engine. Though barely over twenty, he thought of a new way to handle the fuel and the air that, mixing together, exploded to thrust the plane forward. When the new engine was given its first big secret test, Cal was the one to pull the throttle. Success! A thrill he still recalled vividly years later. This resulted in his first patent, although it belonged to General Electric.

Later Cal liked to say we both fell in love at the same time, that first night we talked to each other at the holiday party. I never agreed. Love was too big a thing for me to have it happen that fast. But maybe he was right. All I know is once I let myself love him, I was never able to stop.

I went to Mexico for my divorce. My oldest daughter, Susan, now in college and on winter break, came with me. I hated the sleazy town. The vulgar ceremony. The loud laughter, the dancing in the streets, the cardboard signs stating in bold color, "Welcome to Freedom!" and "Celebrate!"

I almost left. I felt ashamed. I still do a bit, now. But I think it shows how special it was to be loved by Cal, how much I was willing to go through to be with him. Before I met him, I remember sitting in front of my dressing table on my thirtieth birthday and crying. I was so disappointed in myself. I hadn't managed to write anything but an article about twins for a magazine, and a few poems. I hadn't even graduated from college. I felt like a total failure except for my children. But somehow, by some kind of magic, Cal and I found each other, having missed in both Tenafly and Poughkeepsie, and the world changed. Less than a year after my divorce, I married Cal and began the wonderful years of my life.

We were married in a little church in Franklin Lakes, New Jersey, at eleven o'clock in the morning on June 25, 1969. We invited only our parents and our children and our minister and his wife. Both sets of our parents were in their eighties and frail, so they opted to send gifts rather than attempt the long drive. Six of our seven children were there (Cal's oldest son sent a congratulatory telegram from California, where he was working hard as a physicist).

It was far from a conventional wedding. The church was banked with flowers, not for us but rather in preparation for a funeral scheduled to be held that afternoon. I wore a short white silk dress that Cal had helped me pick out. The minister, a longtime friend, escorted me down the aisle before performing the ceremony. Joan, Cal's oldest daughter, played the wedding march on the church organ while Karen, Cal's youngest daughter, took pictures. Later, at the wedding brunch in a country inn, our children raised their glasses in a toast.

Karen drove us to the airport, where we caught a plane to Bermuda. It was my first time there, and I thought it was the most beautiful place I'd ever seen. As well as beautiful it was clean, so clean it seemed as if it had been scrubbed each night and then put out to dry the next morning.

We were there for a week. Memories flood back: swimming in the ocean each morning before breakfast, making love, riding bicycles built for two, laughing.

Cal wanted me to play tennis, which he loved. I said I couldn't, because I could only really see out of one eye, remembering failed Ping-Pong games with my father as a little girl. "You can," Cal said. "I'll teach you. I don't want anyone else as my tennis partner the rest of my life." He was far, far better than I was. But he patiently volleyed with me and taught me how to hold my ground at net so that, later, we could play as a team.

Cal insisted on wearing socks on the beach so his feet wouldn't get sunburned, and I kidded him about that. For his part, Cal never let me forget that I asked what altitude we were at in Bermuda, as waves washed against the shore just inches from where we sat.

Chapter Three

B ack in New Jersey, our honeymoon officially over, Cal gave
up his New York apartment and moved in with me. It was
an easy move. The year before we married, I had rented an
apartment in Ridgewood, New Jersey, a town close to the school
where I was teaching. Our children were now away at college,
so we just pushed together the two maple spool beds my mother
had had made for me when I was a little girl, bought some king-
sized bedding, and squashed my clothes over to half the closet.

We wouldn't be there long. We couldn't go back to Tenafly. Our divorces, followed by our wedding, had shocked and
scandalized our friends. Almost no one we knew had left their
spouses. So instead, we had put down a deposit on an apartment
high in a building under construction on the New Jersey side of
the Hudson, close to the George Washington Bridge. But for
the first stretch of our marriage, we happily shared my small
rented one-bedroom only a few miles from where I taught.

Since the early 1960s, I had been a volunteer and then a teacher
at a private school for seriously emotionally disturbed children.
I worked from eight thirty to three thirty helping them with
communication, relationships, and academics.

I had never planned or even thought to be a teacher. But

someone had suggested that volunteers might be needed at a nearby school for children with emotional problems. So, as placement chairman for the women's group I belonged to, I went to investigate.

The morning I visited, the children and teachers were having "Circle," their opening exercise, marching around a big room while the director thumped out "A Farmer in the Dell" on the piano. I felt a deep connection. The place seemed familiar to me; it seemed I belonged. I knew too that I had to work there, and I began as a volunteer.

After three years at the school, I got a call from the director saying one of the teachers had been in a bad automobile accident and was severely injured. She wanted to know if I'd be willing to take over her class. I was horrified to hear of what had happened to the teacher. But willing? Willing to teach every day? I couldn't believe it. I felt as if Christmas, my birthday, and New Year's had been rolled into one and I had been given the gift of a lifetime.

"I'd love to do it," I said. "When do I start?"

"Tomorrow" was the reply.

So, for several years before I married Cal, I drove to a nearby church that let the school use five of its classrooms during the week. On Fridays we packed everything away and unpacked it again early Monday morning. (It would be many years before the school had its own building, a beautiful new place, complete with a swimming pool.) There was one teacher for every four students. My first year teaching on my own I had three boys and one girl. The boys remained with me my second year, now talking to each other, and a new girl joined us. She spent her days in the closet at first. I slowly lured her out.

Halfway through that year, another teacher, Dave, suggested we combine our classes. "I could use your help with my girls, Mary," he said, "and I can help with your boys." When he learned I was taking an evening class at a nearby college in an effort to get certified, he also offered to drive me to it, saying he had a class at the same time.

I knew friendly feelings were all I felt for Dave. Cal and I were growing serious about each other. But I appreciated the ride. So on Thursday evenings I left my car at a parking lot near the highway to the college. Dave picked me up, and then dropped me back at my car later. Each evening when I left, I waved a thank-you and called "See you tomorrow" to Dave.

Little did I know, and not until Cal and I were married did he tell me, that he was there in the same parking lot every Thursday night to watch Dave help me out of his van, and to make sure no kisses were going on.

Cal was working even harder than I in these years before we married. He had one idea after another, all focused on new ways of heating and cooling. One of his first inventions was the Roll-A-Grill, still used in many football stadiums and diners. He'd noticed hotdogs often burned while workers were busy filling drink orders and making change. So he designed a set of heated metal tubes that kept the hotdogs turning while they cooked.

Using webs of plastic tubes with hot or cold liquid running through them, he'd invented a heating pad that could wrap around sore joints more easily than a hot water bottle, and a blanket that could warm people without the danger of electric wires. He even designed a way to keep the Apollo astronauts comfortable in their space suits when they went to the moon.

Not all his ideas fared so well, though. Demand for his biggest early product—a new kind of furnace with small flexible duct pipes, developed out of his work on the jet engine—had soared initially, leading Cal to greatly expand production. But one part supplied by another company turned out to be faulty. Cal replaced the parts but this and a drop in sales left him with huge debts. He was forced to file for Chapter 11—bankruptcy.

Cal said driving down to Newark repeatedly to go to court to sort this all out was the hardest thing he ever did in his life. But he did not give up. He sold the patent on his furnace and a second patent to pay off most of his debts. He then argued he could come up with more ideas to cover the rest of what he owed. The judge was persuaded, and Cal threw himself into a series of new inventions.

So in the first years of our marriage, as in the preceding years, we were both very busy. But we were doing what we loved, and in love with each other.

Chapter Four

M y little Ridgewood apartment was fine during the week. Cal and I both worked long hours, and in the evenings we were so glad to be together we barely noticed our surroundings. But on weekends we felt the need for more room. I was writing, Cal was inventing, we needed space to think. So we began driving up to Yelping Hill.

"Yelping Hill? That's a funny name," I'd said when first hearing it.

"It's called that because of all the foxes," Cal said, explaining how their nightly serenades resounded about the hill.

Cal's father and some other professors and their families had vacationed together for several years, sometimes in the mountains and sometimes at the seashore. But the time came when they wanted a place of their own where they could return each summer. "Couldn't we find a few wild acres somewhere and share expenses and responsibilities?" one of the women had asked. In the 1920s they found a quiet remote spot in the upper northwest corner of Connecticut and bought five hundred acres of land. It was rumored the price was only ten dollars an acre. The group was very proud of their business smarts, saying now no one could call them absentminded professors.

Each family got four acres of land on which to build a house.

They put in a communal tennis court and decreed that the side of the property that edged a lovely lake would never be built on except for docks, floats and two small changing rooms. Aside from an old barn and a few small outbuildings that were still standing, the rest of the five hundred acres would remain woods.

On my first trip to Yelping Hill with Cal, we drove through an open wooden gate, up a rutted dirt road, and before any cottages came into view, there was the Barn, wood-shingled and three stories high, greatly remodeled after the purchase. The front door opened into a large living room with a stone fireplace against one wall. Above the fireplace hung a quilted banner portraying a rather odd-looking fox. Bookcases covered other walls, and at the back of the room a porch looked out over a grassy field filled with lilac bushes and wildflowers. When I arrived in 1969, everyone had their own kitchen, but in the beginning the Barn was where the families ate every meal. Who cooked? Not the women.

The story goes that the husbands asked the wives how they wanted to spend their summers. And they replied, "Painting and gardening, hello-ing and playing tennis, reading and putting on plays, and visiting. Not cooking or looking after the children."

The husbands agreed and hired a group of Yale boys who were free for the summer to live in the four bedrooms on the top floor of the Barn and take care of the children and the meals. The only thing each husband asked for was a small, separate cottage, away from the main house, where he could write and where no one would ever clean.

Everyone built the kind of summer house they wanted; some were small, and some were big. Most had bathrooms and running water, but none had kitchens or electricity. Everyone ate every meal at the Barn, the children with their Yale counselors, the adults together at different tables. After dinner they gathered in the living room and read plays out loud or watched a marionette show put on by the children or square-danced in a separate building called the Hay Loft. They also played games. Cal told me one game of Murder lasted all weekend. The lethal weapon turned out to be a bicycle pump.

Cal's parents built a house that sat high on a hill above a meadow with an apple tree in the middle, a stone fence along one side, and a western view of the sun setting behind the mountains. Cal's father designed the house and then hired an Italian stonemason to build it out of stones dragged up by horse and wagon from the meadow. Cal's parents named the house Fridstol, meaning "Free Chair"—after an old English tradition of a stool in a church. If you could reach that stool, no one could harm you. That's the way they wanted their house to be.

Cal's parents had given him their place more than a dozen years earlier when it had become too much for them. The year before we were married, Fridstol hadn't been opened because Cal had been consumed with rebuilding his company. When we arrived together for the first time, windows were broken, and mouse dirt and more lay across the floors. Cal immediately set to work to get the water and the heat turned on, intricate systems devised and understood only by him.

The house was cold and messy. I stood alone in the huge living room and called to Cal, "What can I do to help?"

"Oh, I don't know. Shake out the slipcovers and vacuum, I guess."

I cautiously approached the couch in front of the fireplace and lifted out one of the seat cushions. There in the seam of the slipcover were bones, the bones of a small skeleton.

Oh, I thought. *What kind of place is this?* But I tugged away, got the slipcover off, took it outside, and shook out more bones. I looked for a washing machine. No luck. I found a broom and dustpan in the hall closet. But then, as I was carrying them across the living room floor, I heard a noise behind me. I turned and saw a fierce-looking animal about a foot long with bared teeth coming toward me.

"Cal!" I called. No answer. I could hear him somewhere in the attic.

I put the slipcover down, climbed onto the bare sofa and from there to the marble checker table that stood behind it. I had never been frightened by a mouse or a bat, but what in the world was this strange wild creature?

Now there were two more of them coming out from the cupboard beneath the bookcase.

"Cal," I called again, helplessly.

And then, suddenly, all hell broke loose. Cal's brother, Jimmy, came up the front walk with his little dog. Jimmy pushed open the front door, and the dog took off after the animals. Jimmy was yelling at the dog, I was calling for Cal, and the animals, which I later learned were weasels, were climbing the stone walls. I barely knew Cal's brother. I felt like an idiot perched on the table.

Cal finally appeared, helped me down from the table, and suggested I might want to take a little walk. I did. *What was I getting myself into?* I wondered. I tried to imagine my gentle mother coming to visit and couldn't. It was dusk when I got back to the house. I opened the door. A fire was burning in the huge fireplace. It was warm. The floor was clean. The weasels were gone.

Cal was waiting. He put his arms around me. "I'm sorry," he said. "That's never happened before. But I hope you'll come to love this place like I do."

And it did become a wonderful place to spend our weekends and summers. But I have to admit to a few doubts in the beginning.

Chapter Five

It seemed to take forever, but finally our new apartment was ready, and it was worth the wait. Twenty-one stories high in the sky, and the sun flooded into the living room through the glass doors that led to a small balcony. At night the lights of Manhattan studded the sky above the Hudson River. We moved in my grandmother's cherry chest and tables, and with the last of our money we bought a king-sized bed and white wool carpeting for the living room.

One day about a week before we were to move in, we stopped by just to check things out. When we opened the front door, we were amazed to see one of the building crew sprawled out on the carpet. He was just as surprised as we were but rose gracefully, spread out his arms toward the sunlight, and said, "Just like the beach!" We repeated that phrase often after we moved in.

Someone gave us a waterbed for the guest room, and for the living room Cal made a large coffee table out of slate, declaring, "Every teacher should have her own blackboard."

We left our apartment each weekday morning in our separate cars—I to teach and Cal for his office in his plant, now renamed CalMac. Our days were packed. Cal had paid off all his debts and was working hard rebuilding his company. I was caught up in my teaching and the notes I was trying to keep about the children I taught.

I worked at that little private school for six years. The salary was small, but I loved helping the children. Somehow, I could hear them even if they couldn't speak, and as they came to trust me, they began to grow, even to learn to read and write. Some were able to move on to settings in public schools.

Then, just two years after Cal and I were married, the director called me into her office to tell me that the school had become accredited, and she could no longer use me as a teacher.

"I'm sorry, Mary," she said. "You're a natural teacher and I'd like to have you continue, but I can't. It's a state requirement that all our teachers be certified. The best I can do is to keep you on as an aide."

An aide? I thought. *After working with the children for six years?* I shook my head. I had those two years at Wellesley, and I'd been taking education courses for years, but night credits accumulated slowly, and I still had a ways to go before I would have the correct initials after my name.

Cal, of course, was Cal. "It's a really good thing. Hard, I know," he said, kissing my forehead, "but a good thing. Now you can go to college full time. You'll have your degree in a year or a bit more at the most, and then you can do anything you want."

I didn't mention how much I would miss the children. They were the warp and woof of my life now that my own children were away at college. But of course, Cal knew this. Instead, I said, "But the money? I know it isn't much, but we've counted on it."

"We'll manage," Cal said. "As long as we have each other, we'll always manage." This was before many of Cal's inventions or my books were successful. I knew he was right, but it was also true that we had very little income.

So, in my mid-forties I went back to college. Few older women were doing so at the time, and I found myself surrounded by fellow students in their late teens and early twenties in a cafeteria overwhelmed by the sounds of The Grateful Dead. But we got used to each other. They were, after all, the same ages as my own children. I learned to keep my mouth closed rather than blurting out advice, and they cheered me on just when I was ready to give up on New Math or swimming twenty consecutive laps. "Sure, you can do it. No sweat," they said. And when I did, they bought a bottle of wine for us to celebrate.

While I was at school, Cal was inventing. Cal often made models of his new ideas, using cardboard and scissors and glue. Sometimes he'd bring these home from the office to show me, or to work on. I loved hearing Cal talk about his work. I didn't understand physics or chemistry, but he was good at describing his ideas simply, and I enjoyed listening to him as he did so.

"See, Mary, metal conducts heat and cold really well," he'd explain patiently, "and plastic doesn't. So everyone uses metal. But plastic has great other qualities. It's lightweight and flexible, and if I run the right solution through these little tubes, they can freeze water quickly and efficiently."

Cal had a big new project he was working on. The plastic tubes he'd used to make heating and cooling pads and blankets could be woven together into something much bigger—a lightweight portable ice rink!

The standard approach was to dig a large hole in the ground and install permanent metal pipes in it, anchored in concrete.

These rinks, laborious to build, sat covered over and unused most of the year.

Cal's ice rinks could be set up quickly and easily almost anywhere, on a tennis court or indoor basketball court, or even the stage of a theater. First some plywood—or, if indoors, a tough waterproof sheet surrounded by low plastic walls—was laid down and covered with a layer of sand. Then Cal and his men would roll his mats of plastic tubes out over this, pump an antifreeze mixture through them, and pour water on top, which hardened into a big smooth sheet of ice. His rinks could be kept frozen any time of year, even in hot summer weather.

Cal had already installed over two dozen skating rinks, and even a toboggan slide. He was caught up in ways to improve his rinks even further.

Experimenting with a new way to freeze ice in one of his indoor rinks, for example, he found himself skating through slush. Initially stumped, he soon figured out the ceiling above him was radiating heat back down to the ice. What to do? He devised a simple lightweight drape that, hanging high above the rink, absorbed the heat instead, cutting the cost of freezing the ice by almost a third.

For my part, though my courses seemed endless and often meaningless, I persevered. Finally, I was awarded a degree in elementary and special education. But then I could not get a job. I had applied for every teaching vacancy in the public schools around me. One place after another turned me down. I think I seemed too old to them.

In the end, I decided that if no one was willing to hire me, I'd just have to create my own job. I'd set up my own practice. This meant shifting from special education. I had loved working with autistic children, but I felt that to reach them I had to be with them all day, in a setting providing additional structure and support. I needed a way to work with children on my own.

I decided to go on for a master's in learning disabilities at the same college. This meant more classes, more exams, and worst, more time away from teaching. Two things saved me here.

First, the psychologist I had known at the school where I'd taught for six years called and asked if I had time to help a ten-year-old who had "school phobia." Then came an acting-out teenager who was barely able to read. I had studied dyslexia and dysgraphia and thought I knew some techniques that would help him. But the psychologist said, "Well, fine, but don't worry about techniques too much. I'm sending him because I know it will help him just to spend time with you. I watched you for six years, you know."

That was one of the nicest compliments I ever received. I began seeing children again, on a one-to-one basis after school in a room at a local church.

Second, the public school system in the small city where I was working on my master's found they had a long list of "socially maladjusted" children and not enough counselors. They turned to the college, looking for students in special education that they could train.

For once, my advanced age worked in my favor. I had experience. I was selected to work with a "maladjusted juvenile delinquent," Luke, who turned out to be a sweet-faced little boy in second grade. Yet he did have quite a record of truancy, and many arrests for stealing and setting over a dozen fires.

One picture from those days is permanently burned into my brain. Leaving Luke's school one afternoon, I found I'd locked my car keys in the car. Frustrated, I kicked the front tire and then got a wire coat hanger from the school closet, bent it into the shape of a hook, and was pushing it through a crack in the car window to pull up the little knob on the car door. Suddenly Luke appeared, followed by two or three other boys. He said, "See, I told you she was okay. She knows how to pick a lock."

I worked with Luke for two years. By the end of our second year together, Luke's "crimes" had diminished, and he was now performing at grade level. On my side, I found Luke and the three other children I was later assigned as fascinating to teach as those I'd worked with earlier. It seemed the switch I was making in my teaching might work out.

But I had not forgotten the autistic children I'd taught for six years. They remained vivid in my mind. I had kept notebooks during my years at that little school, writing about all the things happening there. What I really wanted to do now, audacious as it seemed, was to turn my notes into a book.

Chapter Six

Four years into our marriage, Cal and I were both happily immersed in each other and in our work. Nights and weekends were spent together and with one or more of our own children. Weekends we'd head for our house in the country.

Encouraged by Cal, I was taking my writing seriously, trying to make progress on my book. On weekend mornings and in the summers, I retreated with a mug of coffee to scribble away, filling page after page of big pads of paper. I liked using these because I could write freely, knowing I could rip out and crumple up whatever seemed awful later.

While I wrote, Cal, when not repairing something on the Hill, worked on his inventions. His mind was so active, his head always full of ideas. Cal loved developing his own products. "I'm a problem-solver," he'd announced more than once. He'd often tell me coming up with a new idea was just the beginning. Being willing to persist until the project worked was what mattered most. At times Cal would have to admit defeat when an idea just didn't work. But when he finally succeeded, he exulted. "I did it! I really did it!" he'd crow to himself, and later to me. It was almost like falling in love, he said.

At Yelping Hill, Cal often sat in the living room sorting out his thoughts and making drawings in one of the red spiral-bound notebooks he always had with him. He always jotted down all his ideas for inventions as they evolved, joined with sketches of how they looked. Every few days he had another engineer read through his notes and initial them. This proved useful when he applied for patents, showing clearly that he had come up with his ideas himself.

In the evenings, before dinner, he would show me what he'd been working on, and I would read what I had written that day to him. He always loved every word. "I can't wait to hear what you write tomorrow," he'd say.

We found Yelping Hill such a productive escape that we began going up even on winter weekends, although the stone house was designed only for summer. Often the snow lay six inches deep on the ground, but we had the local garage clear our road, and we holed up in the back part of the house. Our water supply was in the attic in ten big new garbage cans that Cal had wrapped in insulation and filled from the Hill's tank before it was drained for the winter. Connected by improvised pipes to those in the kitchen and bathroom, the water flowed down easily when we turned on the taps. Cal's furnace heated the rooms we used, and its flexible ducts, running along the top of the walls, could be pulled down to dry wet hair or heat up our cold bed before we got into it, snuggling together under his hot water blanket. Surrounded by Cal's inventions, warm and cozy, we were happy.

What made our relationship so very special? First, we were so glad we had found each other. Maybe we had learned how rare it was to find the right person. I felt treasured by Cal, and I think he felt equally loved by me. Also, at the heart of our relationship was a very strong desire to help and support the other, joined with a belief each could succeed.

We had a genuine interest in each other's projects, even though we did such different things. I knew nothing about engineering, and Cal had never taught children. But we truly enjoyed hearing about each other's days and new thoughts and experiences.

Friends often teased us at Yelping Hill. We'd come down to the lake to swim after working all morning but end up talking intensely to each other instead. Cal would get caught up in hearing about how my writing had gone, or I'd be intrigued by some new piece of his latest invention.

I finally received my master's in learning disabilities. I was thrilled my college days were over! But I knew I had to get a teaching job and establish contacts before I could set up my own office.

Yet, once again, no one wanted to hire me. After all that education, the only position I was offered was that of a teacher's aide in one of the public schools. I seemed to be "over-qualified" for anything else. I suspected this was, again, a polite way of saying "too old" to be starting a public school career. I still didn't want to be just an aide. But I took the job.

Then one day I received another call from the psychologist who had referred children to me. He told me of a nearby school that was looking for a part-time person to run their resource room, where children with learning disabilities received individualized help with reading, writing, and math. He urged me to apply. I did.

Amazingly, I was offered the position. Finally, I was in charge of my own school room again. The psychologist had said, when telling me of the job, "It will work out well as you build your practice."

I hoped he was right.

I took another step forward. I had always dreamed of having

my own office, and I finally found a small space in an old house converted to a professional building. I shifted my one-on-one sessions with children after school there.

Most important, I finished what I hoped was a book about the autistic children I'd worked with for so many years. But I was afraid to let anyone see it. Cal was encouraging. He helped me find an agent, who then sent out my manuscript. Nervously, I waited. It came back rejected. My agent sent it someplace else. It was rejected again. And again. More than six times! Cal remained calmly certain I would succeed.

He turned out to be right. One day I learned a big well-known company wanted to publish what I had written! In 1974, my first book, *Circle of Children*, came out.

Cal was having his own successes. He was even more productive than I was. His plant was working efficiently, manufacturing and marketing his inventions in heating and cooling technology. Mark, Cal's youngest son, had finished college and joined Cal's firm. Things were selling well. Cal's inventions were beginning to attract attention once again. While I was writing about the children I worked with, others were writing about Cal.

His IceMats were appearing all over the place. They intrigued people. A number of newspapers and magazines carried stories about him. Reporters were fascinated by skating rinks that could be set up on gym floors and parking lots, or even float on top of swimming pools.

Rockefeller Center installed one of his IceMats. An increasing number of universities and towns were also doing so. Cal's invention was revolutionizing the way skating rinks were built, becoming the new standard in such construction.

Mary MacCracken

———

Cal didn't stop there. Always thinking of new ways to do things, he was already involved in several other exciting projects. He was filing one patent after another.

Cal was exploring ways to use his mats to heat as well as freeze, coming up with an early solar hot water panel. From the start of his career, Cal had seen the potential of solar power. He'd actually been interviewed on television in the early 1950s, saying we needed huge arrays of solar collectors to capture the sun's energy.

Again, Cal turned away from the heavy combinations of metal and glass that others commonly chose. Instead, he used plastic tubing again, laid out in black mats that, exposed to the sun, could heat up water in homes or even swimming pools. SunMats, he called them.

Chapter Seven

As both of us succeeded more and more in our work, we began to think of buying a house. We had left our high-rise apartment after two years, renting half of a duplex closer to Cal's plant and my work. Now, though, we were drawn to having a place of our own.

We found a wonderful house nestled into a wooded hill in Englewood that an architect had built for both his family and his office. It had two bedrooms and baths, a fireplace, and over the garage, a big room I too could use as an office. It was only a five-minute commute to Cal's plant and, with the children I worked with coming to my house, none for me. Also, with the move came a change of wardrobe. No more suits and heels. Instead, jeans, bright sweaters, and sneakers, which the children I worked with liked even more than I did.

Our dinners were late now. We had a drink in the kitchen while I cooked a simple meal. We lit the candles on our dining room table and talked all through dinner. We enjoyed the details of each other's day, both the successes and errors. We even offered each other suggestions, though our fields of knowledge were far apart. This, in a way, was helpful because we had to describe what we were doing without using any technical jargon, and it made our own definitions and decisions sharper and clearer.

We were never critical of each other. We only had one or two fights. Once Cal was driving me to a photographer's studio to get pictures taken for use in my new book. The man lived somewhere near our place in the country, not far away, he'd said, though he was rather vague about how to get there. We made an appointment to stop by on a Friday afternoon before reaching Yelping Hill. We found ourselves on endless country roads without signs, winding around and around, running out of time. I was anxious. Cal refused to stop and ask directions. I finally lost it. "Stop!" I yelled. "I can get there faster myself!"

Cal pulled over, I stormed out of the car, slamming the door behind me, and marched off down the road for almost a mile. Cal drove slowly behind me, finally coaxing me back into the car. We did find the photographer, eventually. We weren't even late.

But we rarely fought, and we didn't just work. We also had fun, not only kidding around with each other but playing tennis with friends, going to parties, and traveling. The increasing success of Cal's inventions took us to places like England, Germany, Switzerland, and Brazil. We were happier than we'd ever been, and more in love.

Once before we were married, I'd said to Cal, "You know what I would like? Just once I wish you would write me a love letter."

"Okay," he agreed easily.

Cal was an engineer, a very creative engineer, but still an engineer.

When my letter arrived, it began, "How do I love you? Let me count the ways." A neatly organized list followed: # 1 _____ #2 _____ #3 _____ #4 _____ and so on.

But despite his poetic limitations, he gave me so much. He believed in me, encouraged, almost dared me to do things I would never have thought I could.

One day, the president of the National Mental Health Association called and said he'd read my book, *A Circle of Children*, and his board was interested in fostering more interest in children's mental illness. Buzz Aldrin, the astronaut, was just finishing his term as honorary national chairman. Now they wanted to invite me to be the honorary chair for the coming year.

Me? National chair? I'd barely been out of New Jersey, and I'd never done any public speaking. I thanked him as best I could but said I really couldn't. I had a contract with a public school and a practice I was very committed to. He urged me to think about it, but I declined.

When Cal came home, I told him about the phone call.

"That's wonderful," he said. "You'll be great."

"I turned it down. Cal, I've never done any public speaking. I thanked him, but I said no."

Cal smiled. "That's no problem. Just call him up tomorrow morning and tell him you've thought about it and would like to accept."

"But, Cal, it sounded like all the past chairs have been famous."

Cal said, very seriously, "Mary, this is your chance to help emotionally disturbed and learning-disabled children all over America. Just because you're scared doesn't give you the right to turn that down."

The next morning, I called and accepted the position, still wondering how I'd ever do it.

My principal agreed with Cal and said he'd find a substitute to cover for me when I had to travel. I found another trained teacher who could work with the children I saw in my office while I was gone.

My excuses erased, I entered one of the most exciting years of my life, traveling down to Washington, DC, for board meetings and across the country to speak at mental health lunches and dinners. I was always nervous before I began, but I did love teaching and helping the children become more successful. Once I started telling their stories, I forgot to be scared.

Cal would always pick me up at the airport when I returned from each trip. We'd collect my suitcase, and he'd settle me into the seat beside him. Then as he drove me home, he'd sing, corny as it sounds, to the tune of "Hello, Dolly," "Well, hello, Mary, yes hello, Mary, it's so nice to have you back where you belong."

And I'd think, *I'm never going to go away again.* Of course, I did.

Cal was making great strides in his own work. He had come up with another way to cool things. On hot days everyone wanted air conditioning, and this put an immense strain on power plants. Instead, Cal thought, why not freeze a big block of ice during the night and then draw from it during the day to cool the building? He was using plastic again: big plastic tanks to hold water and small plastic tubes with coolant in them to freeze the water during the nighttime and then carry cold from the melting ice block into the building during the day.

This idea would become his biggest success. It was called thermal storage: storing cold in ice during off-peak hours and using it during the daytime. The electricity used in freezing the ice cost much less during the night, when far fewer people were using it. His system saved hospitals, schools, businesses, and apartment buildings a great deal of money.

———

Our monetary fortunes were increasing. Demand for Cal's off-peak air conditioning system, as it came to be called, was rapidly growing, and my first book was being made into a CBS special starring Jane Alexander. Cal bought a new building in which to manufacture his ice tanks. I was starting another book.

Cal was still playing squash, as well as inventing, and succeeding there also. He won the sixty-and-over national squash championship twice in a row, giving him almost a dozen national championship wins in all.

Not everything went well. Just a few days before Christmas one year, the building Cal had just recently bought caught on fire and burned to the ground. We were up all night watching the flames.

But once again Cal didn't give up, was not daunted. He saw this as a chance to focus on the inventions that mattered most to him, those tied to his off-peak air conditioning. His big tanks of ice, frozen during the night to cool buildings during the day, were selling all over the world. One evening Cal came home to tell me he'd just gotten a call from someone high up in the military in a Middle Eastern country.

"What are these ice tanks you are building?" the general had demanded angrily. "Why are you selling these tanks to our enemy?"

Slowly, carefully, Cal had explained.

My second book about working with troubled children got published, and then a third. I then found I wanted to write about some of the children I'd been working with privately, and that book got published also.

Cal's ice tanks, now called IceBanks, were a great success,

and he was getting one patent after another. Soon he had almost eighty! A well-known business magazine featured him on their cover, calling him "one of America's most prolific inventors." A big publishing company asked him to write a book for others about how to develop, patent, and sell their own original ideas. "An inventor," Cal cautioned in it, "must be willing to fail repeatedly, to risk scorn and bankruptcy." He himself had certainly done so. But he had persevered and succeeded. With his help, so had I.

It was a shining time. For the first twenty-five years of our marriage, the world just shone. So many good things happened during those years. We both wrote and published. Cal invented and created and sold. I taught and spoke to groups across the country. We walked in a haze of happiness.

"Duck soup," Cal had told me once the year before we married, "the rest of our lives will be duck soup if we ever get out of this mess," referring to our failing marriages, our painful divorces, his battle with bankruptcy.

It seemed he'd been right and that we were set for life. We loved our work, we loved each other, we relished our evenings together. Our house was a happy place, full of ideas and affection.

"We'll stay here forever," we promised each other. "When we get too old to work, we'll retire and roll around in our wheelchairs. We'll have someone live up in the office space who will cook and take care of us—and not mind that we're still in love."

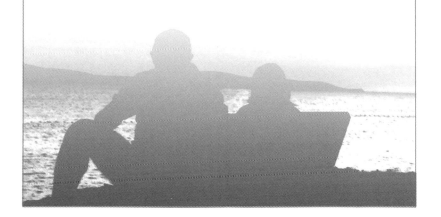

Part II

EARLY
ALZHEIMER'S

Chapter One

Then, slowly at first, our life together began to change. In the beginning it was just little things. Cal started to lose his ability to spell. This didn't seem important to me. Many of the engineers Cal worked with couldn't spell either. Cal had simply started carrying a small dictionary around with him to look up words.

There were other small signs. He began to get lost driving to places we'd often visited. Refusing as always to ask directions, he'd say, never sounding worried, "It's just around the corner," and he'd finally reach where we were going. He had increasing trouble finding his keys and glasses, but we all do, I'd thought. He learned to always put them in the same spot and developed a series of other routines to help him remember things. He set items he wanted to take to work with him right in front of the door so he couldn't miss them.

Cal also did things he'd never done before, but these also didn't seem too serious. One evening I heard his car arrive and the overhead garage door bang shut. I knew he was home, but he didn't appear. I went to investigate. I found him still standing in the garage outside the door into the kitchen with his keys in his hand. He shook his head.

"I can't figure out which one unlocks it," he said. We painted the key red with some old nail polish of mine, and he never had trouble again.

There were also small funny incidents. When we were in Englewood, we slept late on Saturday mornings and then lingered over breakfast. On one of these mornings, I told Cal that a friend of ours, Marcia, had called and asked if we'd like to have supper with her and her husband and then go with them to see a new movie, *The Scent of a Woman*, that evening.

Cal sipped his coffee and said, "Sure, sounds good."

Later that afternoon, coming back in from raking leaves off the terrace, he asked, "What time are we going to see that *Smell of a Girl*? We laughed about that.

None of these seemed major issues.

Things had also changed at Yelping Hill. We were no longer in the big stone house designed by Cal's father. It sat on a sprawling piece of land, a mixture of meadows, slabs of granite, stone walls, and pine trees, with a view of mountains in the distance. For twenty years we had spent as much of our summers as we could there, and after our tumultuous first visit, I had come to love the big five-bedroom house almost as much as Cal did. Most of the year we could only go up on weekends, as both of us were working hard. We set off early Saturday mornings, or sometimes the night before, stopping for dinner on the way. Cal drove. He was a good driver and he enjoyed it, whistling as he got behind the wheel. I always had a book with me, and most times I read out loud.

It was just a two-hour drive from our home and work in New Jersey, but there was no trace of suburbia. Cars were trucks or aging Volkswagens, and occasionally a station wagon or two. Most clothes were jeans and faded T-shirts, boots, or sneakers, the older the better.

Everyone on the Hill worked in the mornings, writing, painting, or doing repairs. In the afternoons we played tennis and swam in our communal lake. Evenings were spent at the Barn for potluck suppers, talk, and games.

Cal and I worked, played tennis, and sometimes saw friends in the evenings. Often, though, we chose instead to stretch out on the couch in front of the fire, reading and talking to each other about what we'd done that morning. Dinner could come later.

Then, in 1990 or so, Cal had proposed giving the house to his sons. Knowing how much Fridstol meant to him, I was surprised. But there was another small house on the land, originally Cal's father's writing cabin, called the Domski. Cal hired an architect to turn it into a little house just for us. He referred to it at first as a guest house, then suggested we try it out. I didn't even suspect a disease called Alzheimer's then. We kept the original one-room cabin as our living room with its stone fireplace, heavy wooden doors, and peaked roof. We added a new kitchen and dining area, a couple of bathrooms, and one big bedroom. "One bedroom is all we need," Cal insisted. "There are five other bedrooms down in Fridstol. Family and friends can stay there."

We had seven children between us, plus some spouses and thirteen grandchildren, so Fridstol often had a jumble of people of all ages, with much noise, confusion, laughter, and sometimes quarrels. Cal, generally patient and friendly to all, had been getting worn out and irritated by the chaos. Later I realized that it was not the kind of atmosphere that would have been easy for an increasingly confused brain, but at the time I thought moving out of the big house was just another of Cal's new ideas. He'd always had some project or other that excited him. Looking back, I could see there had been other hints that I hadn't noticed, or maybe deliberately ignored.

The Memory of All That

Others were noticing, though. Cal's youngest son, Mark, worked down at the plant with his father every day and had done so for almost two decades. He was now also taking over the care of the big house at Yelping Hill, spending many weekends there. One morning when Cal was off on an errand, Mark came by to talk to me about how Cal was doing, asking if I'd seen any changes. A little confused sometimes, I told him, a little irritable, but still as loving as ever.

Mark told me of incidents at the office. Cal's longtime secretary was the first to notice, upset a couple of years earlier by Cal's failure to make a word plural. "This is the only time in my twenty years here that he's misspelled anything," she'd exclaimed.

While this was minor, mistakes at work had grown. Cal was misplacing items and losing track of what he was trying to say to the engineers he worked with. Recently, he'd failed to recognize a visitor he'd just had a long talk with a few days earlier.

I listened. I thanked Mark for his concern. *Maybe Cal is no longer perfect*, I thought to myself, *I still love him*. But I did begin to wonder what was going on with his brilliant mind.

Shortly after that, Cal's oldest daughter, Joan, who was a doctor, called. She urged me to get Cal to see a neurologist. "If we find out early enough what the problem is, there may be things that can be done," she said.

That November 1992, feeling maybe a vacation and escape from daily pressures would help, Cal and I flew to Bermuda to celebrate his seventy-third birthday. We'd gone there on our honeymoon, walking the beaches in a cloud of love and joy, so it seemed the perfect place. Back then we had stayed in a tiny inn, as we couldn't afford more. This time we chose a bigger, fancier place. We walked the beach in the morning, played tennis with friends in the afternoon, but made reservations for dinner for just the two of us.

We dressed up. We held hands all through dinner. We walked back on the beach to our hotel room. But I had begun to worry that Cal had a tumor inside his beloved head, small at first but growing larger every day.

"Darling," I said, "would you do something for me? Would you come with me to see a neurologist? It's probably nothing, but your children and I are a little worried about you."

Cal did not speak to me the next day or the next. It was as if our twenty-some years of being joined at head and heart had vanished. We ate meals together, even played tennis with each other and friends. But Cal didn't talk to me.

Instead, he sat on the small terrace outside our room and wrote on one of the yellow legal pads he always used. I sat beside him and tried to read, my eyes filled with tears, wishing only that I could take back the foolish, inadequate, awkward, stupid words I'd uttered.

Joan was right. Cal did need to see a doctor. But why hadn't I been wiser and found a better way, a different place to talk to him about all this?

The day before we left, Cal asked, "Would you like to hear what I've written?"

I nodded, for the first time in our life together leery of words.

Cal read me a long letter that he had composed, recounting his many accomplishments of the past year, the speeches he'd given, the committees he'd chaired, and a few business deals he completed.

When he finished, he turned and looked at me. "How does anyone think there's anything wrong with me? I do not need to see a neurologist or any other doctor."

We flew home the next day. I doubted we would ever go back.

That winter we went to spend Christmas with Joan and her family up in Maine, as we'd done for the last several years. Joan and her husband, also a doctor, had two children, and Cal was relaxed and happy to be with his family.

It was the perfect place for Christmas. There was always snow, sometimes coming down in big white flakes the size of pennies, and a tall brightly decorated tree inside. For Christmas Eve, their traditional meal was lobster, fresh Maine lobster with melted butter, which Cal and I had always found a special treat.

The evening started well. Cal and I were warmly welcomed into the cheerful house and sat enjoying our drinks by the fire while the others bustled about finishing preparations for dinner. We all sat down at the table. Joan's husband, Bob, gave us each a lobster and began to help me crack the shell and pry out the meat from mine.

Then I heard a grunt from Cal, who was sitting across from me. He had picked up the whole lobster in his hands, shell and all, and was biting determinedly at the claw. No success. He turned it around and bit hard again.

"Here, Cal," said Bob calmly, quickly shifting over to his side, "let me help you with that." He worked away, extracting all the lobster meat onto Cal's plate and then taking the empty tails and claws away from both of us. Cal accepted his gentle approach, and dinner went on without fuss, full of stories and laughter.

Later, though, Joan took me aside. "Mary," Joan said, "you've got to get Dad to a neurologist for an assessment." I knew she was right. I said I wished I knew how to find someone knowledgeable I could trust. She promised to do some research and come up with a recommendation for us.

After the holidays, Joan, keeping her promise, called with the name of a doctor widely considered to be the best. I suggested to Cal that we go see him, not an easy conversation. As in Bermuda, Cal resisted, continuing to say he didn't need to see a doctor. He really didn't want to go.

But inside he must have known something was wrong, and somehow, he finally found the words to talk about it.

Chapter Two

We were up in our little house in the country. It was still early spring. Purple violets covered the ground beside the gray slabs of granite, pale pink flowers burst out on the wild azalea bushes that grew in the woods, and the songs of birds surrounded us. We were the only ones at Yelping Hill. Our summer community of friends had not yet started coming up. But we couldn't bear to be there for just a few months of the year. This was where I wrote, and Cal sketched and sorted out his ideas for new inventions.

It was cool but not freezing, so we could have a fire in the evenings in the living room, and we loved going in there after dinner to read and talk. I was sitting on the sofa reading under a lamp. Cal was lying stretched out with his head in my lap, half dozing. Then he began to talk, so quietly at first I could hardly hear him.

"I'm scared," he said. "I don't think I've ever been scared in my life, but I am now." He sat up, and I moved close to him and clasped his hands in mine.

"Something's wrong," he continued. "You know I can't spell anymore. I can't figure out how much tip I should leave, so I just write down anything. I forget all kinds of things. Sometimes I even forget where I am. I don't know what's happening to me."

I turned to hold him closer. "We're getting older, Cal," I said gently. "We'll be okay. We have each other, and together we can handle anything."

Cal unwrapped my arms and kissed my palms. "I love you" was all he said. We sat side by side for a while, holding hands, not saying anything, staring at the fire. But inside, while I was scared too, I was relieved to hear Cal finally admit something was wrong. He had fought hard over the last year to deny what was happening. "Cal," I said, "I'll go to the doctor with you. Don't worry."

But after we went back to Englewood, Cal, being Cal, took matters into his own hands and made an appointment himself with the doctor Joan had recommended, telling me he intended to go alone. One night, though, as we were driving in to the theater, Cal said, "If you still want to come with me to that doctor, it's okay."

"Good," I said, relieved. "What made you change your mind?"

"Because I know you'll get me to tell you all about it," he said, "so you might as well be there."

So in the end we drove together to meet with the specialist, Dr. Winslow. He talked to us both together in his office first. Then he ordered a whole battery of tests for Cal and took him off for a physical. Cal later told me there had been six "student" doctors in the examining room with him, and the head doctor made him take off all his clothes and "poked" at him. He also evidently showed Cal three objects.

When we all met back in his office, Doctor Winslow said, "I told you I wanted you to do something when you came back. Would you please do it?"

Cal looked confused. "You asked me to do a lot of things."

The Memory of All That

Dr. Winslow waited and then said, "I showed you some things. Tell me what they were."

"You showed me a lot of things," Cal said, still looking confused.

"I showed you three specific objects. What were they?"

"Orange," Cal answered.

"Yes. That's right. One was an orange. What were the other two?"

Silence.

After several minutes, Dr. Winslow said, "Never mind. I don't want to embarrass you." He switched to another topic. Over the next few months, an excruciatingly long time for us, Cal was given blood tests, an MRI, and a battery of neurological and psychological tests.

In the end, we were told Cal had no brain tumor, no cancer. Instead, Dr. Winslow, though not the easiest man to talk to, tried to reassure Cal, saying he had mild short-term memory loss. The word Alzheimer's was never mentioned.

Cal must not have been that reassured, however. All the tests and time with doctors, joined with his own fears, apparently led him to feel something serious could be going wrong with him, though he didn't talk about it again. Always a fighter, looking for what he could do in a bad situation, he then applied for life insurance, without telling me. One evening a few weeks later, in the fall of 1993, he brought home the letter from the insurance company.

> "We regret to inform you that we are unable to accept your application for long-term life insurance because of your existing condition of Alzheimer's disease."

Finally, we had a name for what scared us.

Mary MacCracken

———

Despite the awful letter, our lives went on much as before. Cal still drove to work each day and often went to a nearby diner for lunch, as he'd done for many years. His office and plant were only a few miles from our house, and he knew the route well. So I didn't worry about him. I felt I should be doing something, but I had no idea what.

Then shortly after New Year's, a friend, Ellen Sanders, called and said, "We're getting up a table for the winter ball at the club, and we'd love it if you and Cal would join us. We hardly ever see you anymore."

I thanked her and told her I'd check with Cal and get back to her, but I was hesitant. At the last cocktail party we'd attended, Cal got everybody's name mixed up and then was embarrassed and upset. I didn't want to put him through that again. While there would only be a small group at our friends' house before the dance, there would be a mob at the club. But when I talked to Cal about it, he was enthusiastic. "Why not?" was his reply. He loved to dance, and at our age we usually just danced with the person we came with, so maybe it would be all right. And it would be fun to go to a party again.

So one wintry evening, Cal donned his tuxedo and I put on a long green evening gown with spaghetti straps. We viewed ourselves in the hall mirror before putting on our coats. Cal grinned and said, "Not bad for a couple of old goats."

After cocktails with a group at Ellen and Jim's house, we went on to the club for dinner and the dance. Everything was okay so far. Ellen had remembered that Cal had once done a commercial for Ballantine ale, and he was pleased when she handed him one to drink.

Inside the club house, a cheerful crowd milled around the

dance floor. Many shook Cal's hand with genuine warmth; at one time he had been president of the club for several years. He smiled back, and I was glad we'd come. But when we gathered for dinner, I noticed with surprise and some trepidation that there were eight place cards set out around our table. I found mine, but Cal wasn't next to me. Instead, Ellen had placed him across the table between her and Stacy, a blond newcomer to our group.

Uh-oh was my only thought.

But it was too late to change anything. It would only cause a fuss and call attention to something that might never happen. My dinner partner, Ted Plover, was an old friend. We'd gone to dancing school together, and his best pal was my first boyfriend. Ted's wife had died the previous year, and I wanted to tell him how sorry I was and hear how he was doing.

Cal and I danced a few dances, Cal moving across the floor as gracefully as ever. Back at the table, Cal settled himself beside Ellen. All seemed to be going well. Ted turned toward me.

"I'm glad to have a chance to talk to you, Mary. Thank you for your letter about Beth."

"Your wife was a wonderful person," I replied. "I know you must miss her terribly." I knew this was not the most appropriate place to talk, but I wasn't sure when we'd get another chance.

"She was in a lot of pain . . ."

"Mary," came a shout from across the table. "Look at Cal. Look at what he's doing!" shrieked Stacy.

I'd been watching Cal closely, but when Ted began talking about his wife, I'd become engrossed and forgot to keep an eye on him. Now I could see that Cal had picked up his piece of pecan pie with his fingers and was happily munching away, crumbs tumbling down his cheeks onto the table. I wanted to shout back at her, "So what?!" But, of course, now the whole table was staring. I got out of my chair and over to Cal as quickly as I could. Passing Stacy, I badly wanted to jostle her arm, spill a bit of the coffee in the cup she held onto her silver dress. I didn't. Instead, I touched Cal's shoulder.

He stood up beside me at once, still holding the pie. I said, as calmly as I could, "How about one more dance before we go?" Anything to get us out of there. For a minute, I thought Cal was going to bring the pie with him, but he took my arm with his other hand, hesitated, then put the pie back on his plate and led me to the dance floor.

Five minutes later, I waved our thanks to Ellen and Jim, and we were on our way. That was our last big party. We were quiet on the ride home. Cal was driving, his hands steady and his reactions quick. No sign of confusion. How could he change so quickly? Confused and unaware just minutes ago, aware and competent now. I didn't understand. I knew I needed help for both of us. The same old questions. But who? Where?

Chapter Three

Her name was Nancy Dubler, and it was her help and guidance we needed. I didn't know her well, but I knew about her. She and her husband, Walter, had bought the somewhat tumbledown, welcoming house up the road from our place in the country. Walter was a professor at a college in New York. Nancy was a lawyer who worked in medical ethics, guiding patients and family members through difficult medical decisions. She had written several books, including one about Alzheimer's and was known for her big heart as well as her mind. In the summer, Walter and she would come down to the lake late in the afternoon, and before she swam, she'd float on her rosy plastic raft gazing at the sky and projecting calm across the water. She currently worked as an ethicist at a well-known hospital in New York.

I knew she would know a lot about Alzheimer's, and I knew she liked Cal. I thought maybe if I could get them together, Cal might open up and ask some of the questions I had no answers for. I called her secretary and set up an appointment. The only thing I worried about was telling Cal. He had told me many times how much he hated going to Dr. Winslow, having to undress in front of a crowd of young doctors and be poked and prodded. But when I mentioned to Cal that I had made an appointment with Nancy Dubler so we could find out more about Alzheimer's, all he said was "Okay."

Nancy was all I had hoped for and more. Cal asked questions: "What causes it? . . . Will I die? . . . What's the worst thing about it? . . . Can I still play tennis?"

Nancy answered each one slowly, without condescension. "No one is certain what causes Alzheimer's," she said. "They think that plaques and tangles build up, especially in the regions of the brain important to memory, but there is still some question as to what causes them and why they're there. A great deal of research is going on right now. It's good you discovered your Alzheimer's early on and will be able to take advantage of this research."

"And no," Nancy continued, "you probably won't die of Alzheimer's. In fact, you're in such good shape I don't think you'll die of anything for quite a while. And you'll be playing tennis for years, certainly longer than I will."

An hour later as we put on our coats and prepared to leave, Nancy handed me a card. "Call this man. Dr. Stevenson is a neurologist I know personally. He's brilliant and he's kind. You'll both like him."

On the way home Cal said, "That was a lot better than that doctor we saw before in the city, don't you think?"

Silently I blessed Nancy. Out loud I answered, "Absolutely. A one-hundred-percent improvement."

I called Dr. Stevenson the day after our visit to Nancy Dubler and was given an appointment a few weeks later. Cal went reluctantly, but Dr. Stevenson was in the waiting room to greet us, and Cal willingly followed him into his office. They returned after about forty-five minutes. Dr. Stevenson thanked Cal and then said to me, "Your turn now."

The Memory of All That

His office was warm and a little cluttered. Piles of papers stood on his desk; pictures of lakes and sunsets covered the walls alongside his framed credentials. He offered me a chair and then took the one behind his desk. I studied him in silence—sandy hair, smile, wrinkles around his blue eyes, young, probably in his forties or early fifties. He broke the silence.

"I understand the diagnosis of Alzheimer's has already been made. I concur with that and . . ." He paused. "I'm so sorry. I did give Cal the mini-mental test. If he weren't ill, I think he would have scored over the top. As it is, he struggled to remember answers, not always successfully."

I could feel the tears welling in my eyes. *I will not cry*, I said to myself. Out loud I asked, "What can I do?"

"Try to be as patient as you can. He will become more and more dependent on you. Unfortunately, there really aren't any good medications at this time. None seem to help much, and some people get mean side effects. You need to know it's not going to get any easier."

We talked for a few minutes more, though I don't remember anything we said. Then Dr. Stevenson escorted me back out to Cal and bid us both goodbye. I wondered if Cal felt as helpless as I did. Neither of us said anything. Cal just reached for my hand as we walked back toward the car.

Without plan or suitcase, we drove straight to the Domski. Actually, Cal drove till we stopped to pick up something for supper on the way, then I did the last bit. We agreed we'd just stay overnight, leaving the next morning.

Our little house was a pleasure, warming up in just a few minutes. We didn't turn on the lights. The candles and the fire in the fireplace were enough.

We went to bed early and slept close together, although I dreamed I was riding on the wings of a skylark, high in the sky, circling over our meadow.

Cal was already up and dressed when I came out from the shower wearing yesterday's clothes. He gave me a morning kiss and then said proudly, "I clapped the trap."

I looked at him; he was smiling, but what was he talking about?

"Good," I said tentatively.

He swung out his arm and pointed to the fireplace. "Clapped the trap," he repeated.

Now I got it. He'd closed the chimney damper.

In spite of what we had learned, once home we continued in our routines. Cal drove his old station wagon to work each day and to his favorite diner for lunch, as he'd done for many years. I felt he was safe. His secretary sat just outside his office, and his son Mark was also there each day. When summer arrived, we enjoyed time together at Yelping Hill, where Cal still played tennis as skillfully as ever and liked seeing old friends and family.

Cal did grow more dependent on me. He wanted me around as much as possible. He loved going grocery shopping with me, as this was something we could do together. He would push the cart down the aisles, and I would select items or suggest he put one or another in the cart.

Cal also began to come home from work an hour or two early some days. He confessed to me that when he did so, he liked to sit on the bottom steps of the stairs to my office and just listen.

"Why?" I asked. "Why do you do that?"

"Because it always sounds so happy up there," he explained.

The Memory of All That

——

But the doctor's diagnosis, though gently put, confirmed what we had feared. Cal truly had Alzheimer's, an irreversible degenerative disease of the brain. Having faced it ourselves, it now seemed time to tell the children. His daughter Joan, having helped many families in her work as a doctor, suggested this would make Cal realize he had nothing to be ashamed of and that his family was supportive.

Cal bravely agreed to this plan. We invited everyone to Yelping Hill to celebrate both Thanksgiving and Cal's birthday, his seventy-fifth, which was the following day. We spent the first day cooking and then eating around the big dining room table at Fridstol, which stood at the back of the large front room. It was a lovely meal, with a fire going in the big stone fireplace and the sun setting behind the mountains at the end of the long meadow to the west. The next evening, we gathered again, eating turkey sandwiches and watching Cal open his presents. Then he stood up, took a big breath, and said, "I have something to tell you all. I have a touch of Alzheimer's."

His children were supportive, talking over each other. "We love you just the same," said one. "That's okay," another called out, "I think my memory's going too, Dad."

Joan gave him a birthday card in which she'd written memories of a few things they'd done together when she was younger. Cal's face lit up. He could remember each of the events and add details his daughter had forgotten. Overall, it seemed to make things easier for him to tell his family what was happening.

Still, the disease was relentless. Language was getting harder for Cal. He hesitated as he searched for the word he wanted or substituted another if he couldn't find the right one. Often the first part of a sentence would come out clearly, like, "When we get to . . ." but then drop off to a mumble. Sometimes I could guess what he wanted to say, and I could fill in for him, adding "Yelping Hill" or "We need to call our friends Jean and Edward," and Cal would nod and say, "Good idea."

But often I didn't have any idea, and the unfinished sentence would just have to dangle there.

Although Cal still went to his office, his work, which had always been a great joy to him, was not as gratifying as before. He came home one night and said, "It's different. People used to stand in line outside my office to talk to me. No one comes now."

Dinners, which had once been such a pleasure, where we told each other our ideas over long candlelit meals, were full of awkward silences. I brought a small television into the kitchen where we now ate, suggesting we watch the news, which Cal had always enjoyed.

Weekend mornings, once a time for long talks and cuddling, were awkward now also. I told Cal I thought it would be fun to go out to breakfast. So on Saturday mornings when we didn't drive up to the country, we began going to the local diner. Creatures of habit, we soon ordered the same thing each week: orange juice, coffee, toast, and eggs, over-easy for Cal and poached for me. We enjoyed being waited on and starting the day slowly.

But I didn't always handle things well. One afternoon Cal got mud on his shoes and then tracked it all over our white kitchen floor.

"Oh, Cal," I sighed, "wipe your feet." I probably shouldn't have said anything.

He was furious and stormed off to get the vacuum cleaner. I said I thought a sponge would work better. Again, I probably shouldn't have.

"Don't tell me what to do," he retorted, then vacuumed for ten minutes.

When I went into the kitchen to make dinner, the floor was still dirty. I didn't say anything, for once, just washed the floor with a sponge. Cal ate a big dinner, as always, and the next morning said he had slept well that night. I hadn't.

Changes could also create problems rather than solving them. In our Englewood house we each had our own bathroom. My old scale had malfunctioned, and I bought a new digital one. One morning Cal wandered into my bathroom, stood in front of the scale, and said, "Can you show me how this thing works?"

"Sure," I said. "See this little black tab on the front of the scale? You just touch it with the tip of your shoe, and three zeroes show up. Then you step on the scale, the zeroes fade away, and your weight appears. It's kind of neat."

Cal said, "Okay. I get it." He stepped forward, slamming his foot down on the tab, which broke off. "Why do you always set me up to fail?" he yelled and stamped out of the room.

I picked up the broken scale. Words tumbled through my head. *Set you up to fail! That's the opposite of what I try to do.* I tried to remember what I'd read. *It's not Cal talking. It's the disease!* Still, my heart cracked a little.

Chapter Four

I didn't know what to do. I felt like I was losing Cal, but some-how it seemed disloyal to tell anyone else about it, at least anyone who knew him. Then one evening I saw a notice in the local paper announcing that an Alzheimer's support group was meeting at a nearby hospital at one o'clock on Wednesday after-noons. The hospital was only twenty minutes away from our house. My first student on Wednesdays didn't come until three. I had given up all my work in the schools and was doing only private practice in my own office now.

Cal was still going to his office every day though. He had just made his son Mark president of CalMac and himself CEO. I knew Mark would be there at the plant and I could go off on my own in the afternoon.

The following Wednesday after lunch, I set out. I easily found the hospital, a large, sprawling building. I started down the hall, my footsteps echoing behind me. I heard voices com-ing from behind one of the doors, and I opened it as quietly as I could. I'd arrived a little after one o'clock. The meeting had already started, but everyone stopped talking and looked at me.

A woman who seemed to be the leader said, "Can we help you?"

"Is this the support group for Alzheimer's caregivers?"

"Yes. Are you a caregiver?"

"Yes."

"Well, welcome. Come join us. My name is Carol. What's yours?"

"Mary," I mumbled as ten pairs of eyes stared at me. There were two men and seven women plus Carol.

One man cleared his throat. "As I was saying, we just can't get her to take a shower. Yesterday when the helper was there, we tried. But even with the two of us, one on each side, we couldn't get her in."

Carol said perhaps his wife was frightened. She suggested getting a hose with a spray attachment so the water wouldn't come directly down on her head, and perhaps a stool that she could sit on.

Would this happen to Cal? I couldn't believe it. We both enjoyed our morning shower. Cal whistled as he soaped and rinsed, and I loved to hear that.

The next person said she'd had a good week. She'd found that if she read poetry out loud to her husband, it reduced his pacing and wandering. The woman next to her asked how she could keep her husband from putting potatoes in his coffee. Carol suggested a container with a cover, like the mugs used for traveling.

I wanted to leave. I liked Carol and thought her suggestions were helpful, but this must be another disease. This wasn't Cal. I just couldn't imagine him doing any of these things. This couldn't, wouldn't ever happen to us. I wanted to walk away, but I had already interrupted by arriving late. I couldn't leave until the meeting was over.

Carol stopped me after the meeting. "I have a feeling that group might not be quite right for you. How long has your husband had AD?"

AD? That must be short for Alzheimer's disease. Oh, there was so much I still had to learn.

Quickly I brought my attention back to Carol. "We've known for over a year. But I think we all, including my husband, suspected something before that." By now I'd realized that things had been different for quite a while.

"Do you have any family or friends to help you with this?"

"We have seven children between us, but the only one near is Cal's youngest son, Mark, and he's very busy with work. Cal just made him president of the company he founded fifty years ago. And I don't think Cal would want me to talk to any of our friends."

"Look," said Carol, "I have a free hour right before this meeting. We could meet in my office down the hall, just the two of us, if you'd like."

So began my meetings with Carol, and they did help. I can't remember what we talked about now. Only that those Wednesday afternoon visits were very important to me, though much of the time I said little, as tears that I kept inside everywhere else poured down my cheeks.

But I was bothered by the fact that Carol wouldn't accept any money from me. She said she couldn't. She was paid a salary by the hospital, and it would be unethical to accept any other money. She was so good, so knowledgeable and kind, that I had to do something. One day she invited me to go with her to the Alzheimer's Day Care room where she worked every morning. There were about a dozen people in that section, a mixture of men and women, and, as I was slowly beginning to understand, many different degrees of AD.

The patients were bussed in every morning, stayed through lunch, and were then picked up in the late afternoon and bussed back home to their spouses or other caregivers. On this morning they were all sitting around a large table with two attendants, molding bowls out of clay. Some bowls were quite elaborate, complete with handles and designs; some were rudimentary; and some nonexistent as the supposed bowl-makers dozed in their chairs. In the background, scratchy music came from a somewhat battered portable record player. *Now I know what I can do*, I thought. *I can buy a new radio and CD player for the Alzheimer's Day Care Center and give it to Carol.*

I did, presenting the gift to her just before we moved away. This move was also due in part to Carol, for she helped me take the next step—a huge one. Talking to her, listening to others in her support group, and dealing with Cal's growing problems had led me to realize I couldn't care for him alone. I needed lots of support, more than an appointment with a doctor or weekly meetings with a social worker, however good. I needed a whole network of care. I began thinking about how to arrange this for Cal, and for myself as well.

Then a friend opened up a new path I'd never considered. Every Tuesday morning for several years, except during summers, I had been driving into New York City, which was not far from Englewood, to meet with five other women, all writers. Over the years we had helped each other with our writing. Now, one of them, Natalie, helped me figure out how to best handle the time ahead with Cal.

"Mary," she said, taking me aside after one meeting that spring, "I've found a wonderful place for us to grow old. It's a CCRC, a kind of retirement community that will care for us the rest of our lives, called Kendal at Hanover. I'll tell them to send you some literature."

A CCR what? I thought. I'd never heard of such a place or thought about going into a retirement home. But Natalie, as well as pretty and fun, was very bright and perceptive. Though she never said anything, I knew she was aware that something was going on with Cal, and I trusted her judgment.

The literature arrived and I read it all carefully. Kendal was located in Hanover, New Hampshire, and was called a CCRC, meaning a continuing care retirement community. It provided several types of living arrangements. We could start in our own apartment but then shift to assisted living or a nursing wing if needed. It was one of a handful of non-profit retirement homes started recently by Quakers. Pictures showed lovely low white clapboard buildings set out in the country, and the floor plans of the apartments were appealing. It seemed to me a genuinely good place. It cost a fair amount of money, but it meant we would never have to move again, and we would always be together under the same roof.

Cal wouldn't even look at the brochure. "I'm not going into any retirement home!" he announced firmly. But I knew I couldn't let it ride. Once we had dreamed of spending our old age in the home we loved so much, rolling around in our wheelchairs. Now I thought of us growing more and more isolated alone in our house. I'd learned I couldn't handle Cal and his growing needs by myself. Cal had always prided himself on being a problem-solver. This time it was my turn. I would find a way forward for us. A retirement home with good health care seemed the answer.

In the following months, I made appointments at several different retirement homes in the Northeast, and Cal and I went to see each of them. None felt right. At most places people dressed up a lot for dinner. Everyone, though elegant in appearance, seemed stiff and formal, very different from the casual style of Yelping Hill, or the jeans and sneakers I wore when working with children.

I grew discouraged, and for once Cal was not supportive of me. Driving down to see a place near Philadelphia, lost, hot, and tired, I suddenly felt Cal's old station wagon, which he loved and refused to give up, lurch and then go *bumpety-bumpety-bump*. A flat tire. We were far from any place, out on a small, deserted road. Once Cal would have changed the tire cheerfully, whistling as he did so. This time I had to call roadside assistance. Fortunately, Cal, always intrigued by new inventions, had a mobile phone in the car. We waited a long time, but finally a young man pulled up, removed the flat, and put on our spare tire, and we resumed our trip.

Unfortunately, on the return trip, Cal's old car lurched again, followed by another series of bumps. A second flat tire! Another call for help. The same young man appeared. He quickly replaced the flat with a new tire he'd brought, and we made it home at last. But I almost felt like giving up.

Not Natalie, though. Some months after the brochure from Kendal arrived, having given me time to get used to the idea of a retirement community and visit other places, she called. "It's supposed to be a gorgeous fall weekend, and so I've reserved two rooms at a motel in Hanover. We'll have dinner at Kendal, and you can see it for yourselves. Oh, incidentally, when we were there before, I met a woman, Polly Bunting, who said she'd gone to Vassar and knew Cal. Maybe that will help . . ."

I mentioned Polly Bunting to Cal. He was immediately alert. It seemed she had been his friend when his family lived on campus. "I was only ten and she was a junior in college," Cal remembered, "but she said she missed her younger brothers."

Cal's reservations disappeared. He was all for a weekend visit to New Hampshire, eager to see an old friend from childhood. Polly Bunting had gone on to be a very successful college president herself, and I wasn't sure she would have time for Cal. But it got us going.

Later, as we drove toward Kendal, Cal explained Polly had taught him to band birds. "I slept out on our porch sometimes and made a little house out there to catch birds," he recalled. "I could open and close its roof with a string tied to my big toe." These were a lot of words for Cal.

"Sounds like one of your first inventions," I said, patting his leg.

It was a long drive. Cal was careful about keeping within the spced limit, and we didn't reach Hanover until about four o'clock. As soon as we arrived at our less-than-elegant motel, I looked up Kendal's number and left a message for Polly Bunting that Cal MacCracken, nicknamed Caddy, would be coming to Kendal for dinner and would like to see her.

As soon as we walked in, I loved the place. Everyone seemed self-reliant, happy, and friendly. Polly sent a message to our table: "Let's meet in the living room in front of the fireplace after dinner. I'd love to talk with you."

Polly was a short, compact woman with a gencrous smile, probably in her mid-eighties. She embraced Cal, and they immediately set off on a round of reminiscences about bird banding and early morning hikes. I eavesdropped with pleasure and then asked Polly questions about Kendal.

She said she'd been there for five years and that it was the best decision she'd ever made. The residents were delightful: bright, active, and lots of fun. She also said the medical care was top notch: a clinic, an assisted-living section, and a skilled nursing unit all right there at Kendal.

I also knew the Dartmouth Hitchcock Mcdical Center was just a couple of milcs away. This was familiar territory for Cal. One of his inventions, off-peak air conditioning, was installed in the hospital. Cal himself and a small crew had put it in several years before, and Cal was proud he had done so and that it was still working well.

The next morning, we had a quick tour of Kendal. Cal said, "I think I like this place. I don't know about you."

Me? I thought it was wonderful. Maybe we could handle Alzheimer's. My hopes soared. But all I said was "I like it too. A lot."

We filled out a formal application before leaving.

Chapter Five

B ack home, even with Alzheimer's an acknowledged part
of our lives, our days went on much the same. When the
alarm went off at six thirty every morning, I tried to drag
myself from my dreams. Cal got up, put on his bathrobe and
slippers, and made the coffee. Then he walked to the end of the
driveway, picked up the *New York Times*, and brought the paper
and the coffee back to bed, a daily ritual I found endearing. For
the next half hour or so, we drank our coffee, read the paper,
and commented on the ways of the world, although now Cal
dozed more than he read.

Without really noticing, though, I was doing more and more
for Cal. When we got up we stood on each side of our king-
sized bed and pulled up the sheet, blankets, and comforter. As
soon as the bed was made, we headed for the shower, and then,
while Cal shaved, I laid out two piles of clothes on the bed, one
for Cal, one for me.

Lately he'd been having trouble getting dressed, not sure
what to put on where. Sometimes a shirt went on top of a
sweater. So I laid out his clothes in order. On top were under-
pants, then socks, pants, shirt, shoes, and finally a sweater or
jacket. I tried to stack my pile to approximate his. If there wasn't
time, mine was just a jumble. But I was always nearby so if Cal

put the wrong shoe on the wrong foot or had trouble buttoning his shirt, I could help unobtrusively.

We ate breakfast at the kitchen table. Then Cal kissed me goodbye and left for his office. I put our few dishes in the dishwasher and climbed the stairs to my office to prepare for the day ahead. I wondered, though, how long we could go on like this.

For my seventieth birthday in June 1996, Cal gave me a can of bug spray. I was surprised—startled, really—because in the past my presents were usually jewelry or extravagant clothing. The year before, on my sixty-ninth, it was a diamond bracelet.

Bug spray scared me. But I smiled. "Thank you, darling."

Cal smiled back. "I got it for you because I know you like to work in your garden and the bugs bother you."

Later that month, we decided we'd try to get away from Alzheimer's and go to Russia with a group of Cal's Princeton classmates. Our trip started off well. As we stood in line waiting to board our plane for an overnight stop in Helsinki, an attractive uniformed woman approached us and asked us to please follow her. I immediately wondered if, like the insurance company, someone had reported to the airlines that we had Alzheimer's. But, of course, I knew this was foolish, and we followed silently.

What they wanted was to move us up to first class. Why, I'm not sure, and our friends teased us about bribe money, but we didn't care. We just reveled in the luxury. Wonderful wide seats, sparkling white linen napkins, and wine glasses. We couldn't believe our luck.

Helsinki, a stopover, was a very clean and wonderful city and we enjoyed walking its streets, although our stay was brief.

We boarded the plane for St. Petersburg early the next day. I was a little nervous as we deplaned in the afternoon. It was the first time we had traveled with me in charge of the tickets and carry-ons. I also had to keep Cal headed in the right direction. But the plane landed smoothly, and our group headed for customs. Everything seemed to be going well until all of a sudden Cal shouted, "They're stealing our luggage! Look, see, there it goes!"

He pointed at a large cart filled with suitcases, the driver leaning on its horn to clear a path through passengers. Cal began to run after the cart yelling, "Stop! Stop!"

Three of his friends ran after him. Cal had been a leader at Princeton and his friends followed him even now, joining in with shouts of "Stop, thief! Stop!"

Oh no, I thought. Obviously, it wasn't a thief. The driver was in uniform and wouldn't be honking his horn and calling attention to himself if he was doing anything illegal.

Cal's friends soon came slinking back, and one of them mumbled to me, "They're taking our luggage to customs."

"Where's Cal?" I asked.

"He wouldn't come. We tried to get him to, but he was arguing with the driver."

I trotted off as fast as I could, still holding our carry-on luggage and paperwork.

In the middle of the airport waiting room, a small crowd had gathered around the luggage cart as Cal and the driver yelled at each other in a mix of English and Russian. I wasn't sure what to do. I pushed ahead until I was next to Cal. "It's all right," I said. "He's going to the same place we are."

Cal looked at me in disbelief. I leaned against him and shouted at the driver, "Slow," pumping my hand slowly up and down. Turning to Cal, I said, "We'll walk beside him and make sure he's going to the right place."

A small lie. I had no idea where to go and only hoped the driver did.

I handed Cal one of the carry-ons. "Please help me. They're getting so heavy."

Finally, we collected our suitcases and made it through customs and onto the bus to our ship. When we got to our state room, I collapsed on the bed.

"What's the matter?" Cal asked, not unkindly. "Are you tired?"

We spent four days in St. Petersburg, guided by a charming young Russian man, visiting museums and churches. Never have I seen such large museums or so many churches. Or maybe it just seemed that way because I worried about losing Cal. Somehow, he always got interested in something in the wing opposite the one to which the guide was headed.

There were no more scenes, only now various wives would corner me and say something like "Cal looks marvelous. The youngest of the bunch. But he doesn't talk much. Is he all right?"

When I told Cal about their concerns, he said he didn't want to tell them he had Alzheimer's yet. Family was one thing, friends still too big a step. He did try to talk more, and he danced up a storm every night before we went to bed.

Our ship took us to Moscow. More museums and gold-crowned churches. I told Cal I was having a good time, a second lie. I was very tired and longed to get back to familiar places.

On our last night aboard ship, we had another crisis. This time it was me. I turned on the new hairdryer I'd bought especially for the trip and without warning blew out all the electricity. I was very glad to get home.

Mary MacCracken

———

Back from Russia, we settled into our summer routine. Cal still played tennis well and enjoyed seeing family and friends at Yelping Hill. Everything was very familiar to him, and he liked the relaxed pace of his days.

Then, unexpectedly, in the middle of the summer a call came from Kendal asking us to come to Hanover for a series of interviews. Applicants were usually admitted fairly quickly, within a year or two, perhaps as this retirement community was new, but we'd only applied the past fall.

Cal resisted. He was reluctant to leave our happiness even for a short time. I reminded him that out of all the retirement homes we'd seen we'd liked Kendal the best and that it was important to keep in touch with them. Besides, I added, I was sure his old friend Polly would be eager to see him again.

It was then I began to realize I was shading the truth more and more to make things easier for both of us. Long ago, we'd promised we'd never lie to one another, but that was before Alzheimer's entered our lives.

"It's too soon. I'm not ready yet," Cal said.

"We won't stay," I promised. Actually, I wasn't that eager to go myself. I'd heard about the assessment interviews. Seven meetings in one day, including those with the executive director, the associate director, the social worker, and the clinic personnel.

Cal remained adamant that he wouldn't go.

But Mark and Mike, Cal's two sons, were visiting Yelping Hill, and they took their father off for a walk, and obviously a talk, because when they came back, Cal had agreed to the trip.

The Memory of All That

Fortune smiled on us. At our very first interview, a small gray-haired woman was introduced as a member of the resident admissions committee. She shook our hands and then looked directly at Cal.

"Didn't you have Miss Candee for kindergarten?"

"Yes," Cal replied. "But how did you know?"

"Because I had her too," she answered. Her name was Mary Keeley, and she had indeed been in the same kindergarten class as Cal in Poughkeepsie, over seventy years ago. Under my breath I said a silent thank-you.

Cal was wonderful during the rest of the interviews. As soon as we arrived for each meeting, he would introduce himself and shake hands firmly, saying, "I may have a little bit of Alzheimer's, you know," as if to explain any shortcomings he might have. This, combined with his great smile, worked very well. To top things off, when we were leaving and one of the directors started to look up the parking slot we'd been told to use, Cal interrupted. "It was number 73, I think," he said.

He was exactly right. They were impressed. So was I.

Shortly after we returned to Yelping Hill, Kendal called, saying we'd been accepted and offering us an apartment. It seemed several people had turned this apartment down, though, as it faced north and never got any sun except for an hour or so in the summer. It sounded dreary to me as well. I thanked them and said we'd wait for another unit.

Two weeks later we received a letter from the admissions committee confirming that we were officially accepted. But it also stated that if we delayed too many months, they would ask that Cal have another physical examination. I put down the letter and went for a long walk.

I thought of the bug spray Cal had given me for my seventieth birthday, the strain of trying to keep an eye on him in Russia, and, based on what I'd learned at the Alzheimer's support group and my meetings with Carol, what lay ahead.

I really did not want to give up our life and our house in Englewood. I really, really did not want to lose Cal, any part of him. But I *was* losing him, a little more each day, and as good as he was at trying to cope, things were becoming harder and harder for him. I'd always said, and written in my books about the children I'd worked with, that having a safe place was important. Now both Cal and I needed a safe place. One where he could be cared for by me, but with help from others as things progressed, and where we could stay close to each other.

When I came back from my walk, I went directly to the phone and called the admissions office at Kendal.

"Is the apartment you showed us still available?" I asked.

"Yes. It's being painted" was the reply.

"We'd like to take it, then," I said. I hung up. I could only hope I'd done the right thing.

My call to Kendal, though hard, was only the beginning. Next, I had to tell Cal. Then we'd have to find the money, a lot of money, to pay for the apartment. The entrance fee was a sizeable lump, particularly hard before we sold our house.

But the decision seemed right to me. We could be together in our new apartment, and if eventually Cal had to go into the healthcare wing, we would still be in the same building, and I could be with him anytime, day or night. I couldn't bear to think about Cal being in some nursing home and me all alone in our house.

Two days later I told Cal what I had done. He was very resistant at first. But then he agreed to go there for me. "I liked that place," he admitted, "but we don't have to move in right away, do we?"

Later that day, after tennis, getting ready to take a shower, Cal put his arms around my shoulders. I leaned my face up to his and asked, "How come you love me?" I wasn't looking for a compliment. I only wanted to know.

I was surprised by his response. He put his hands under my chin and said, "I don't just love you. I cherish you." It was so nice he still had such words in him and chose to say them to me.

The next day I got out our dictionary and looked up *cherish*.

Cherish: "to hold or treat as dear—to sustain and nourish something or someone with care, especially in order to promote, increase, or strengthen it."

I copied out the words so that I could remember them and take them with us when we moved.

We were very fortunate in being able to go to a place like Kendal. If we hadn't, I would have taken many steps to build a world of support—a therapist for me, an aide or day care program or both to help Cal when he could no longer go to his office, a doctor nearby specializing in Alzheimer's. I would have confided more in friends, who I know would have offered to help. But it was a relief to think that much of this network had already been put in place for us.

Initially, though, it was a wrenching move.

Part III

KENDAL
AT HANOVER

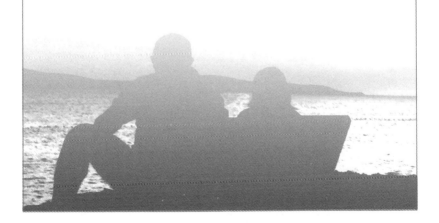

Chapter One

At the end of that summer, 1996, we stood in our newly painted Kendal apartment. We owned it now—paid for and delivered. Home? How could we ever think of this small barren place as home? It seemed a long way off.

Cal walked to the window and looked out at the wide grassy tree-lined square between our apartment and the ones across the way. "No parking lot," he said. "Good."

I said nothing. I missed our Englewood house, our bedroom, my bathroom, my office, my work. Why had I put up half the price (Cal furnished the other half) to come to this place? I shook my head at myself. Not the right attitude. What could I do to make it seem better? Make tea? No tea. No pot. Invite people in? We didn't know any people, except Natalie and her husband Frank, and they were away. No place to sit.

"We need a bed," Cal said in a firm tone.

I moved to stand beside practical Cal. "You're right. Let's go buy one."

We bought not only a bed—well, not quite a bed, a queen-sized sofa bed—but also a wooden card table and two matching chairs with blue woven seats. We put the sofa bed against the longest wall in the living room, a couch by day, our bed at night. Later, when we lived here full time, we'd move it into our second bedroom, which we'd use as a den, guest room, and writing room for me, and we'd buy a new king-sized bed for us.

"Better," Cal said, and it was.

But we had not let go of our old lives in Englewood, despite the six-hour drive between the two places. We were both still working, though much less than in the past. I saw a few children; Cal went into his office a bit. I think of that period, over a year in the end, as an in-between time. Sometimes at Kendal in New Hampshire, sometimes in our house in Englewood, never really here nor there, although we were getting to like the here, Kendal, better than the there.

Kendal at Hanover had grown out of an idea at an annual meeting of Quakers in Philadelphia over two decades earlier. The goal was to provide care for some of the aging members. A grant got the first Quaker retirement community going in Pennsylvania, and a few more followed in nearby states. Ours was the farthest north. We knew winter would come early and last long. But we were happy to trade warm weather for a way of living that resonated with us. Neither Cal nor I knew much about the Quakers, but we liked their basic ideas, especially that there was some good inside of everyone and that the inside was more important than the outside.

This was certainly true of the residents we met, though not all were Quakers. Everyone seemed kind and friendly. Still engaged in many projects, they were more interested in hiking or discussing ideas than dressing up for dinner.

Entering Kendal, I felt a mixture of relief and sorrow. I was glad that Cal would always be well taken care of and that I would have help in meeting his needs. But the thought of how much I was leaving behind—our wonderful home, my office, my students—brought sadness. Would I ever work up here, in New Hampshire? Probably not. I was seventy years old and there was Cal, who I still loved with all my heart and who needed me so much now.

At Kendal, though, we were no longer in a world of just the two of us, as we had gradually become in Englewood. There I had begun to feel more and more isolated. Here many hands were reaching out to us.

On our first night at Kendal when we went down to dinner in the dining room, the hostess led us to a table where a nice-looking man sat alone.

The hostess said, "This is Bob Schaefer. Bob, I'd like you to meet Mary and Cal MacCracken, new residents."

Bob stood up, put out his hand, and then suddenly retracted it. "Not *the* Cal MacCracken, the squash player?"

Cal nodded, smiling.

"Good Lord, I'm an inveterate squash player. I've been reading about you for years. I can't believe I'm about to have dinner with you."

Cal glowed. He tried out his favorite new line. "I've got a little bit of Alzheimer's," he said. It seemed telling his family this the previous Thanksgiving had been a good idea. He didn't feel ashamed or that he had something to hide. I stayed quiet, waiting to see how people we met here would react.

"I know all about that," Bob replied calmly. "My wife had it for seven years." I appreciated his response to Cal. But I also wanted to ask, "Where is she?" I didn't. Maybe because it would have been awkward. Maybe because I didn't want to know the answer.

We were invited to be part of a newcomer's group, as were all the other people who had bought apartments during the last six months. Not everyone joined, but we did, along with five or six other couples and a single man and woman.

A young social worker doing an internship at Kendal had come up with this idea, and she summoned us to a pretty meeting room at nine in the morning on the first Monday of each month. She soon had us discussing the difficulties of moving, as well as the advantages and pleasures of Kendal.

Cal loved this group, and we made sure to be at Kendal each time it met that first fall. He didn't say much, but he delighted in the talk and laughter and friendliness. I was surprised and pleased when Cal introduced himself with what was becoming his stock line: "I'm Cal MacCracken, and I have a little bit of Alzheimer's."

It was hard to believe he had any type of disease because he looked so clean, strong, and attractive. Everyone accepted his statement graciously, and these gatherings soon led to other invitations. One couple, Betsy and Sandy Sanderson, asked us to play tennis, and they became our good friends.

This led to our being asked to join a larger tennis group. Cal and I always started as a team, but after the first set we would switch around, and everyone enjoyed playing with Cal. He was the strongest player there. He reveled in doing something he was still good at, grinning as he put a tricky spin on a return or lobbed over someone's head. But he was also courteous and generous, and he never crowded or took his partner's shot.

Soon Cal wanted to be at Kendal as much as possible. This was also because we had met Dr. Santulli, in his forties or early fifties, dark haired, stocky, soft spoken, obviously bright, and knowledgeable about Alzheimer's. From the start of his medical career, he'd focused on the problems of aging and then come to concentrate on dementia, especially Alzheimer's. He was a gentle, caring man, as well as a knowledgeable one, and he did not talk down to Cal but listened carefully to his questions and answered them all.

Dr. Santulli spent several visits with us explaining Alzheimer's and its components. He suggested prescribing donepezil for Cal. "It isn't a cure," he said, "but it can sometimes slow down the advance of the disease. It's a new medication that's just come on the market—"

Cal, sounding like his old adventuresome self, interrupted, "I'd like to try it." We left with a prescription.

Cal was enthusiastic. "He's great, that doctor. He's the first to do anything helpful." I agreed and understood why Cal wanted to be near Dr. Santulli. Having a doctor who knew so much about the disease and was so good at relating to his patients was a great help.

Cal also loved how friendly everyone was at Kendal. Each person he passed in the halls or on the stairs going down to the dining room would smile and give him a big hello. Cal was also talking more. I didn't know if Cal's increased words were due to the medication he was taking or all the friendly interactions and social stimulation we had. I was simply thankful.

People connected to Cal's past continued to turn up— Beezie, for example. (Her real name was Elizabeth Johnson, but she encouraged everyone to call her by her nickname.) She was a tall woman with excellent posture who, when anyone asked her how she was, always replied, "Splendid," in a most elegant tone. We discovered she had been a student at Vassar during the time when Cal's father was president, and later on the board there and famous for her success at fundraising.

She stopped us in the hall one day and said, "You two have got to come and have a martini with me because . . ." Then she paused and tapped Cal on the shoulder, smiling as she continued, "I know some *terrible* things about your father, and about you too. You were our class mascot, you know."

We all laughed, and then, as we continued to our apartment, Cal said, "I've had some pretty good ideas in my life, but Kendal was the best."

"It certainly was," I agreed, not reminding him he'd sworn he'd never go to a retirement home. Inside I felt great relief. He'd just wiped away any worries I had about urging him to come here.

We began to shift our lives to Kendal. We put our house up for sale. We bought a bit more furniture for our apartment. The living room would do, with the couch and card table, until we moved everything up from Englewood. But we bought two pretty pine bureaus and two nightstands for our bedroom, plus a tall bookcase for all the books I loved. Best of all, though, was the new king-sized bed we purchased from a local store. After it was delivered, we made it up with Kendal sheets, topped by Cal's wonderful invention, the hot water blanket, and a favorite quilt.

We had our new bed set up by dark. After dinner, Cal and I cuddled together under the blanket.

"This is nice," Cal said as he put his arms around me.

"And so are you," I said. "We're going to have a really good time."

Chapter Two

We soon had a routine at Kendal, not perfect but manageable. Cal had always enjoyed making the coffee in the morning, a treat for me also. He continued to do so but now often forgot to put in new filters and coffee grounds, just filling the coffeemaker with water. I thanked him and sipped my faintly brown brew, making a fresh pot later. We continued with tennis, now playing three mornings a week.

We ate lunch in our apartment and every day had a nap afterward. Cal slept and I read, both of us together on our bed. Then we usually drove up the river, the Connecticut River, which ran behind Kendal and beyond. We parked our car in a gravel spot beside the river and walked a mile upstream—we'd measured it first driving in the car—and a mile back, as we'd done from first arriving at Kendal. Cal never tired of it. He loved walking by the river.

Happy with Kendal, Cal started on an introduction to the book he wanted us to write about Alzheimer's. Following an account of his birth, he wrote:

> My mother came to me when I was about three or four, and said, "Calvin, I think it's time you knew how to tie your shoes." She started to tell me what to do, but I said,

"No, I'll figure out a way myself!" This was the first
indication that I would be an inventor. . .

When winter set in, we took on a new activity, cross-country
skiing. The snow, glistening fresh and white in the sun, was
beautiful, and Cal, still a natural athlete, skied easily across a
nearby field. I did my best to keep up.

As the days grew colder and the dark evenings longer, Kendal was proving a cheerful place to be. When we first arrived,
no liquor was allowed to be served in public places. This meant,
in essence, that the place to enjoy it was in our apartments.
Three or more nights a week we were invited for a drink before
dinner to somebody's apartment, or the somebodies would
come to ours, and then all five or six of us would go on down to
have dinner together.

At first, I had a difficult time eating dinner at six o'clock.
Cal and I had always eaten much later because of our work,
but I found that I got used to it and even got to like it. All of a
sudden there was a whole wonderful evening before us back in
our apartment. We put on our warm-up suits, climbed into our
great king-sized bed, and read and read. Heaven for me, and Cal
could doze comfortably beside me. We both loved it.

Being entertained by other people was fun; entertaining
others had its plusses and minuses. Cal and I both enjoyed having
people over for a drink and then eating dinner together down in
the dining room, but preparing for them was another matter.

I laid out wine, scotch and such, cranberry juice, mixers,
and glasses so everyone could make their own drinks, and
then prepared a couple of plates of hors d'oeuvres. While I
was making the appetizers, Cal would start putting the glasses
back in the cupboards. I'd explain they should be left out for

our friends who were coming to visit. But Cal was sure he was helping by picking up and neatening the place before the guests arrived.

Finally, I worked out getting Cal settled in his favorite chair with his Ballantine ale and a small plate of his own cheese and crackers and a timer set for fifteen minutes before the guests, usually just two couples, were to arrive. I told him to stay right there to check if our friends were on time and to turn the timer off as soon as he heard a knock on the door. Unlike in Englewood, Kendalites arrived on the dot of five o'clock. I remember only one time when people were late. The timer went off, but all Cal did was to say, "Uh-oh." The plan worked well, and our friends never inquired why Cal had started eating and drinking ahead of time, or even stranger, why he was holding a timer.

The best thing that came with our move to Kendal was a huge increase in companionship and support. While we had gone to dinner or played tennis with friends in Englewood, even before Cal's illness each of these events had to be scheduled in advance. Here friends lived next door; drinks and dinner, tennis, and other outings were easy to arrange; and we met many people each day in the halls or on the stairs. It was also nice that people were willing to make Cal a part of everything rather than call attention to his differences.

As I was learning again and again, Alzheimer's was too hard a disease to cope with alone. What was getting me through each new stage of Cal's decline was some form of support—wise and experienced people to talk with, like doctors and social workers, but also friends—for me as well as Cal.

The friends we were making at Kendal proved a blessing in many ways. I would occasionally leave Cal with Betsy and

Sandy Sanderson, who'd invited us to join their tennis group, while I had my hair cut or did a quick errand. We often ate dinner or went on short trips together, and he liked them both. But small, simple undertakings involving Cal's care could sometimes seem overwhelming.

One day the dentist who came to Kendal told me that an upper tooth of Cal's was inflamed and probably should be removed. I called an oral surgeon and told him about Cal's tooth and Alzheimer's. He kindly said he understood—his father had had the same disease—and I made an appointment. But then I began to worry. Suppose I needed help getting Cal into the car after they pulled his tooth, or something else went wrong? In a moment of weakness, I asked Betsy if she would go with us. Of course, she said, she and Sandy would both come.

All four of us went into the dentist's office together. We had to wait ten or fifteen minutes. Cal sat quietly beside me as I turned the pages of a magazine, pointing out anything I thought might interest him.

The nurse stood in the middle of the room. "We're ready for you now, Mr. MacCracken." Cal rose. *Should I stay or go with him?* Always new decisions in new territory. While I was still pondering, Cal walked up to the nurse and followed her out of the waiting room.

Cal was gone about twenty minutes. Betsy, Sandy, and I waited. I was too nervous to talk. In my lap I crossed my fingers.

Cal walked back in with the nurse and came over and took my hand. The nurse smiled at Cal and then said to me, "Your husband was a model patient, Mrs. MacCracken."

It was over, just a minor event. Relieved, but feeling silly I'd made so much of it all, I apologized quietly to Betsy as we walked to the car. "It was easy," she whispered back. "We're happy to help you anytime."

Mary MacCracken

———

Years earlier in Englewood I had cut a clipping out of a book review discussing E. M. Forster's writing. I kept it tucked into the mirror of my dressing table. It didn't come with me to Kendal, but I had learned it by heart.

> I believe in aristocracy. . . . Not an aristocracy of power . . . but . . . of the sensitive, the considerate and the plucky. . . . [T]hey are considerate without being fussy, their pluck is not swankiness but power to endure, and they can take a joke.

Was Kendal perfect? No—what place is? But I had found my community of brave and considerate friends. They could also take a joke.

Our first winter at Kendal, some of the residents got together and decided to put on "The Follies." We were asked to be part of it. Cal was in a skit where four men stood on the stage under a fake streetlight singing songs like "Standing On the Corner Watching All the Girls Go By." I was one of the girls. Cal, handsome in his Princeton blazer, whistled.

Later, in the same show, Cal and I were in another skit in which I "bought" a huge pretend cardboard dog at a pet shop. There was an accompanying song, "How Much Is That Doggie In the Window?" and I persuaded Cal to go for a walk with the dog and me. When we got to the lamp post, we stopped, and I was supposed to pull a cord that raised the dog's hind leg. I did. The leg went up. The only trouble was that I couldn't get it down. The audience howled with delight. I tried to drag the dog along on three legs. Cal finally just picked him up and carried him off the stage. The audience roared and clapped.

The Memory of All That

—

That New Year's Eve, 1996, Mary and Jim Keeley had invited us to spend the evening with them. Cal's happiness was contagious. We were both laughing and joking as we dressed for the party, and with happiness came words. I still don't know why this happened, but it was true. If Cal worried about something, his words dried up, but if he was happy and relaxed, the words tumbled out.

We had met Mary Keeley during our first visit to Kendal, when she and Cal realized they had been in the same kindergarten class. Now, over seventy years later, we were celebrating together, the four of us at a table in the big dining room full of many other residents in party hats, elegant food, and festive decorations. Cal and I both enjoyed ourselves. Then dinner was over, and the festivities ended. We were home by eight thirty.

Cal said, "It's too early to go to bed. It's New Year's Eve."

"Okay. What should we do?"

Cal said, "Let's put on our warm-up suits and have a drink."

"Sounds good," I said. But I was alert. Every once in a while, a special awake-time happened for Cal.

There we were, in our warm-up suits, in our bedroom. Cal handed me a scotch and soda and raised his Ballantine ale. "To Kendal," he said.

"I'll drink to that."

"Okay. Now do Mrs. Worthington."

"What?"

"You know, Lady Worthington. That woman you made up for me, after Englewood cocktail parties."

I was surprised. "You remember that? That was quite a few years ago, and that was only for us."

"Well," said Cal, "we're still us, right? Do it one more time."

I sighed, took a sip of my scotch, got out of bed, put one hand on my hip, and said, "Oh, Mr. McLain. No, that's not quite right. It's Macsomething though. So delightful to see you again. Charles, isn't it? And how is that delightful father of yours? President of some place or other, isn't he? Well, never mind. And you, oh, you? On the tennis court, I can just see you. Just gorgeous. I'll never forget it."

Cal turned toward me, laughing. "You are funny, and nobody but me knows how funny you are."

I took another sip of scotch. "That's all I get?" I teased. "For submitting to your request. A weak scotch, and a 'How funny you are.'"

Cal put his arms around me. "Not all," he said, and turned out the light.

Chapter Three

While life was better for both of us at Kendal, it did not stop Cal's decline. We still played tennis, but it began to take all morning now. Matches were scheduled for nine o'clock, but we started getting ready at seven. Everything took twice as long—Cal's shower, breakfast, and particularly getting dressed—at least getting Cal dressed. As I had started doing in Englewood, I laid out both our clothes, but we played on indoor courts, and putting on tennis clothes in the chill New Hampshire winter mornings was new to Cal. He questioned each piece—the white polo shirt, shorts—"I don't want to wear shorts, it's too cold"—even the white wool socks and sneakers. I remembered his earlier doctor's advice, "Try to be as patient as you can." I tried, and once we were on the tennis court, it paid off.

Kendal had a resident doctor, Lizbeth Jones, who also came to be very important in Cal's care. She was genuinely concerned about how he was doing and full of useful information. Helping Cal meant, for me, dealing with a series of small problems on a daily basis. He had lost weight, for example, and Dr. Jones offered advice about what he should or should not eat. She listened to my concerns about changes in his personality—once easygoing and patient, now more stubborn, controlling, and critical. She worked with Dr. Santulli to prescribe and adjust medications to help Cal. I looked forward to my appointments with her. I had great respect for her knowledge and intuitive understanding. It was wonderful to have two good doctors to give me advice.

I also remembered how the social worker leading the Alzheimer's support group back in Englewood had helped me. Lizbeth told me of a similar group in the next town over, and I made myself go. Once again, I found it hard to listen to the problems that others were having with their spouses, all of whom had declined further than Cal. I still couldn't believe this would happen to him. But, as in Englewood, the social worker who led the group, Ruth Whybrow, was wonderful. She listened carefully and was sympathetic. One of the things I liked about her was she gave each of us in the group her own opinion, making clear that's all it was, rather than simply saying, "I feel your pain." She had suggestions for each of us, no matter how perplexing the problem. She became a major source of support for me.

Not everything went smoothly, though. One problem made life harder for both Cal and me. We had put our house in Englewood on the market months ago. But as the end of our first spring at Kendal approached, we'd had no offers anywhere near the realtor's suggested asking price.

Cal grew more and more anxious. "Maybe it will never sell," he worried. "What will we do then?"

The realtor claimed he couldn't understand it. It was, he said, a lovely house with beautiful grounds in a prime location. I also knew, though, that it was old, built in the 1940s, and while it was newly painted inside and out, the kitchen and bathrooms were small and outdated.

I myself had an additional concern. The house, and our going back and forth between Englewood and Kendal, had become entangled with the issue of Cal's driving. Dr. Santulli wanted Cal to stop driving. He had been tested and found to be a "moderate risk" on the road. Cal had always loved being behind the wheel of his car, though. It was the one place he still felt in control, and he really did not want to give it up. I worried. Sometimes, for example, trying to signal a turn, Cal sent the windshield wipers swiping back and forth instead. We worked out one compromise. Cal agreed to split the drive to New Jersey. I then found a roundabout way to the interstate, and when we set out, Cal would drive on the back roads until we reached the highway, then let me take over for the rest of the trip. Returning to Kendal, we did this in reverse.

By now, we both felt it was time to let go of Englewood completely. To do so, though, we had to get rid of all the masses of stuff that filled the big attic and basement of our house. We had lived in our house for over two decades and loved it, and when we bought it, we'd had no intention of ever going anywhere else. Things we no longer needed but couldn't bear to give up, things discarded by our children or passed down by our parents had piled up over the years. The attic was crammed with old pictures in heavy glass frames, a sled, boxes of papers, and bags of clothes. I reassured Cal that once we cleared everything out and got a new realtor, the house would sell, and that we would spend the fall doing this. I wanted Cal to enjoy the summer at Yelping Hill while he still could. I also wanted to go to my fiftieth reunion at Wellesley. Even though I had only attended for two years, I had made good friends and we had all stayed in touch.

Cal was doing so well at Kendal and was so happy and content that it seemed I could actually go away for a few days. Some of our new friends said they would check on him or invite him to dinner, and his children promised to call. He himself, always supportive, really wanted me to see my old college friends. So one warm June day I set off.

I returned just a few days later to find Cal bursting with pride, tired but happy, eager to show me what he had accomplished while I was gone. He had actually driven by himself in his old station wagon all the way down to Englewood and back. He had loaded our heavy wrought iron porch furniture into his car, found his way north again, then wrestled each piece out, into the elevator, up into our apartment, and out onto our little balcony, all without help. "To fix our money problems," he explained, "and bring the larger parts to Kendal."

To start clearing out the house so it could sell, I translated silently, *and bring some of the furniture here*. I was shaken, appalled, relieved he was fine and had not been in an accident. Cal couldn't understand why I wasn't more thrilled to have our outdoor furniture. I did agree to sit in one of the chairs he'd worked so hard to retrieve and have a drink with him on the balcony. But I vowed to sell the house as quickly as possible once summer ended.

That fall, a year after we first stayed in our Kendal apartment, we gave notice to everyone that we were leaving Englewood permanently, and I began to look for a new realtor. Though I appreciated our first realtor's love of the house, Cal was so worried about selling it that it seemed better to drop the price than hold out for all we could get. Cal was eager to help. He made a list of selling points for the house, culminating with #19: "We have lived happily here for 21 years!"

We also tackled the horrendous job of clearing everything out. It was a difficult time, filled with packing and repacking. We had years of possessions to deal with and many decisions to make—what to keep, what to give to our children, what to throw out. It wasn't easy, especially for Cal.

My office over the garage had plenty of deep cabinets that I had filled with the files of more than a thousand children, as well as my materials for evaluating and working with them. Tools, old bicycles, even parts of Cal's inventions cluttered the basement.

Moving was very confusing for Cal. He couldn't under-stand what all the packing was about. He continually unpacked what I had just packed. One day I came down from our big attic and found him on the floor of the pantry surrounded by empty boxes, crumpled pieces of newspaper, and pieces of my grand-mother's Dresden china, which I had just spent some hours carefully wrapping. He held up a creamy white gold-rimmed dinner plate. "Look at the great dishes I just found," he crowed.

After that I kept Cal by my side. We wrapped and packed together and then stored the brimming boxes behind locked doors.

Other things we loaded into the station wagon and distrib-uted to Goodwill or the dump. Cal and the dump man grew friendly. Despite his failing mind, Cal still knew how to posi-tion the car so that the old chairs and broken bedframes we no longer wanted could easily be thrown into the pit.

"There you go," the dump man would shout at Cal as they slid objects from the back of the station wagon into oblivion. "Good job," he'd shout at Cal again as we drove away, Cal smil-ing and waving goodbye.

But, as all too often these days, small triumphs were joined with near disasters. Clearing out the house was hard work, and one night we were just too tired to cook or even go somewhere for dinner, so we called up our favorite Chinese restaurant and ordered take-out.

We parked on Palisade Avenue, a main street, a few doors down from the restaurant. Cal picked up our order, put it in the back seat, got in, started the car, and backed out.

Wham, bam, crash! "Stop!" I shouted. "We've hit something." But Cal stomped on the accelerator, and the car shot farther backward into the street, rocking, then bumping and thumping on one side as Cal tried to go forward.

Cal's plant was just a few blocks away, and I knew his son Mark often worked late. *If I could just get to a phone,* I thought, so rattled I forgot all about the one Cal had installed in the car. I saw a gas station up ahead and beseeched Cal to pull in. Cal parked in the darkest part of the station, but there was a phone booth, and Mark picked up on the first ring. "I'll be right there," he said, after I told him what had happened.

Cal and I waited silently. Mark arrived, told us to leave the station wagon there, and drove us and the Chinese food home, though I can't remember if we ever ate it. Mark came back about a half hour later.

We were sitting at the kitchen table. "Well," he said, "I went back to the scene of the accident, and the truck that was parked next to you wasn't harmed at all. It had a long metal pole sticking out in back, the kind they sometimes use for towing. That's what you smashed into. It made a hole in the back door and the tire of your station wagon.

"Dad, that's the end of driving," Mark said.

I held out my hand to Cal, and without a word, he dropped the keys into my palm. Cal never drove again. I felt sad and thankful at the same time. I knew how hard it was for Cal to lose yet another part of himself. But now it was over. He was safe. No one had been physically hurt. All in all, we had been blessed.

We bought a new tire the day after the accident and a few days later drove back to Kendal. It was raining when we started, but then the sun came out and hopscotched across the puddles. I could feel my heart begin to smile.

Good news had followed bad. Our house had sold. Between giving it to a new realtor and reducing the price substantially, we'd soon had a serious offer. Just this morning, before leaving for Kendal, we had signed a contract and received a down payment. We were promised the rest at the closing at the end of the year. This meant we only had a month to get all of our remaining belongings out, but we could do it. Even better, no more worries about selling the house or Cal's driving.

I glanced over at Cal. He was sitting quietly beside me as I drove. I touched his knee. "See, it's all working out," I said. "I'm proud of us."

"Me too," Cal said and smiled, which made me even happier.

Thanksgiving was a rush of packing and moving last bits out of the house. Our two children who lived closest, Mark and my daughter Susan, came to help. Again, it was hard for Cal. He was helpful, loading up his old station wagon for more trips to the dump, though Mark or I now did the driving. But which things were being saved, which discarded? Cal came upon two suitcases packed with clothes to take to Kendal sitting in the garage near our car. He picked them up and would not let go of them, thinking they should be part of the next trip to the dump. I reasoned with him, getting nowhere. Then Mark approached.

"Here, Dad," he said cheerfully, "let me take those. I know a really good place to put them." Cal released the suitcases at once.

Mary MacCracken

At the end of the day, far too tired to cook, we met at a restaurant downtown for our last Thanksgiving dinner in New Jersey.

A few days later, we drove away for the last time. After we left, the movers came, loaded up the furniture we were keeping, and brought it after us to New Hampshire. Moving our things in was much more fun than clearing them out.

Mark had made a blown-up version of the floor plan of our apartment at Kendal, and I had measured and cut out cardboard furniture, so I knew just where everything should go. The movers, good-natured and thoughtful, let Cal help them move some of the lighter pieces. He loved being useful.

We were all settled in by evening, the movers gone, Cal and I by ourselves now.

Cal reached for me. "I'm glad to be with you," he said.

"I'm so glad also," I replied, hugging him close. "We can be safe and happy here."

Chapter Four

Back at Kendal, though, this time for good, I felt a new upwelling of sadness. I was glad we had sold the house and gotten it cleared out in time. But there was lingering sorrow at leaving so much behind: not just our house and work but friends I'd known since childhood; the cemetery in Englewood where my parents and my brother, Robbie, were buried; so much of my life.

But our world there had shrunk so. Also, it was clear that Cal, and I, needed more support. Little did I realize how hard the months ahead would be and how much Cal would worsen. My optimism would prove naïve. While Cal and I were both safe in our new home, hard times lay ahead for both of us.

We had sold our house just in time. Cal's decline began in earnest. I'd been warned, had seen what others had gone through. But I was not prepared. I hadn't really believed it would happen to Cal. He was going downhill, growing more and more confused. I tried so hard, as hard as I could, to hold on to him, to stop his slide. I couldn't.

At our first appointment with Dr. Santulli that winter after we returned, Cal told me to stay in the waiting room. I knew he hoped to persuade Dr. Santulli to let him drive again. Of course, the answer was no. This was good news for me; at least that worry was truly over. But I also learned that Cal scored much lower on his mental test than he had three months ago. This was a big blow.

Bit by bit, Cal was slipping away. He talked less. I now made the coffee in the morning, bringing it to him in bed. I put toothpaste on his toothbrush. He brushed his teeth and showered by himself. He could still dress himself if I laid out his clothes, working his way through the layers I'd arranged. He still did his chores, emptying the wastebaskets, taking the garbage and recycling to the collection room down the hall, helping do the dishes. We went down to get the mail before lunch. These routines eased him through each day.

But he had increasing trouble at meals. He sometimes poured his cornflakes on a plate at breakfast. Dinners grew difficult as well. He once tried to cut his roast beef with a tablespoon and then eat it with a teaspoon. This took a long time. The couple we were dining with waited patiently. He still enjoyed his favorite dessert, though, two scoops of vanilla ice cream with chocolate sauce.

Cal also started wandering. He went out on three different nights, quietly, without waking me. He found his own way back the first two times. But the third time I woke and went looking for him. A night maintenance man found me before I found Cal and sent me back to the apartment in case Cal had returned home. He hadn't. I waited another hour in the empty apartment until the maintenance man showed up with a chagrinned Cal.

Not having a sense of time anymore, he had gone down to get the newspaper for me. He loved doing this every morning and kept a supply of quarters in a special box on his bedside table so the change he needed was always at hand. But this time he was too early. The papers hadn't yet arrived, so he curled up on a nearby couch and fell asleep. He slept soundly until the maintenance man found him.

The next day all of Kendal was alerted that a photographer would be around to take our pictures, the result of the staff's frustration in searching for Cal with no idea of what he looked like.

Cal could still surprise me, though. Our group of old friends from Princeton, who we'd joined several times for winter reunions in Vermont, wrote urging us to come again, if only for a day. Cal got out the map and then said we could stay as long as we wanted this year, since we were no longer working.

He liked to go shopping at the grocery co-op in town with me. We continued to play tennis with the other Kendal players, and sometimes even won. We went to the exercise room after dinner every other evening to use the weight machines. As our second winter at Kendal finally gave way to spring, known there as the "mud season," we spent more time outside, walking along the river. We still had some sort of life together.

Then one day, Dr. Santulli asked Cal if he would like to be interviewed by one of the big drug companies. Cal was not only willing; he was eager. He did some of the interviews with me beside him and some by himself. He loved it. He had found something he could do that was worthwhile. From somewhere, somehow, he found the words to answer the interviewers' questions. They thanked him and praised him, and that made him very proud.

Cal also learned from the interviewers that the neurological center at the hospital was conducting a research program concerning Alzheimer's. He wanted to be involved in this study. It excited him to think he could be part of discovering new drugs that could slow, perhaps even check, the progress of Alzheimer's.

I was not enthusiastic, but I covered up my concerns because I believed it was Cal's life and he should be able to do what he wanted. Then we learned that Cal first had to stop taking all his other medications, including donepezil, before being put on the trial drug. Cal accepted this with equanimity, but I was worried. Donepezil had really seemed to help Cal.

I struggled. We talked to a doctor at the neurological center, who said that it wasn't known if the trial drug was effective; the study would help determine this. But it was clear that nothing was going to deter Cal. "He will try anything in the name of research," I had told Lizbeth Jones, the head doctor at Kendal, the previous spring. Now Cal was proving me right.

The neurological team welcomed Cal and gave him a long test that involved smelling and identifying different things. It seemed detecting odors might somehow be related to Alzheimer's. Cal eventually grew weary of this and became restless, but cheerfully completed the other preliminary tests and stopped all his medicines.

The doctors said it would take at least four weeks for the remains of the former drugs to be fully gone from Cal's system. This had to be done so Cal's response to the new drug would be clear. Finally, Cal was able to start taking the new drug.

Again, Kendal was a help to me during this time. Residents had turned a stretch of land at the foot of all the buildings, close to the Connecticut River, into a community garden. One woman, no longer able to keep up with weeding and watering, offered me her plot. I knew little about plants, but I began going to the meetings of the gardening group and also found I enjoyed being outside and digging in the dirt.

The Memory of All That

I also made sure I swam once or twice a week. I continued going to the Alzheimer's support group in the next town over.

I watched Cal closely, looking for signs the new drug was working. The nurse at the neurological center said that they had seen some remarkable improvements. One woman who was taking the trial medication was back cooking all the meals for her family just like she used to do. Was this possible, I wondered? Would more of the Cal I had known return?

But day by day Cal grew more confused. He still knew me and wanted to be with me, but he now trembled and hallucinated. Creatures haunted the corners of the room. He stumbled when we walked together down the hall. He could only take tiny steps. He was frightened much of the time. I didn't know if this was due to his no longer being on donepezil or maybe just part of his inevitable decline. It did seem the new drug wasn't helping.

Dr. Santulli said, "This sometimes happens as the disease progresses. Symptoms of Parkinson's disease appear along with Alzheimer's."

He also said, "Maybe it might be time to move Cal to a more structured environment." I assumed he meant some part of the Health Center. But I wanted to keep Cal with me as long as possible. I knew how hard it would be for him to leave, and the thought of letting him go was very upsetting to me.

Some people avoided us now, though I don't think Cal noticed. I didn't really either, until I listened to a plump, gray-haired resident with glasses tell me how she had moved here a year or so ago, and though she had tried, no one wanted to be friends with her. I found this, unexpectedly, deeply sad. I realized I was also feeling sad for Cal, because of the way some residents were pulling away from him as his disease became more evident.

Then we had a particularly bad incident. I now locked us in at night, once Cal was asleep. Not with just the usual lock—Cal knew too well how that worked—but with a special lock loaned to me by our friend Charlie. Charlie told me he had gotten the lock when he was doing a lot of traveling and sometimes had to bed down in unsavory places. It was a strange little gadget about three inches long that slid between the edge of the door and the wall, with a key that snapped it shut. When the door was tightly locked, I put the key in the teapot in the top cupboard, and all was secure until morning, when I unlocked it and put the whole device back in the teapot.

I was reading in the den one evening when the pounding began. I glanced at the clock: almost nine. Who would want to come in now? I went to investigate. Nobody wanted to come in. Cal wanted to go out, dressed only in his pajama top.

"Open it!" he yelled.

"It's shut for tonight."

"Open! Open! Open!"

"Tomorrow morning we'll open it and go for a walk."

"Open!" he screamed once again, and before I realized what he was doing, he grabbed a large knife out of the knife rack and pointed it at me.

Oh, God, what to do? I knew I couldn't wrest the knife away from him. He was still much stronger than I was. I was scared for both of us. I didn't want to be cut or stabbed, and I didn't want Cal to commit a criminal act. I feared if he did so, they might take him away and lock him up in some institution for the criminally insane.

My mind racing, I suddenly realized that not only was he without pajama bottoms but he had no slippers on his feet. I had on my sneakers. I walked up close in front of him. "Give me the knife."

"No!" was the answer.

I gritted my teeth and then, quickly without warning, stomped down as hard as I could on his bare toes.

"Ow!" Cal howled. "Damn you." But he dropped the knife and ran out of the kitchen. I bent down and retrieved the knife and hid it plus the whole knife rack inside the oven. Then I went to look for Cal.

He was lying down, far over on his side of the bed. I lay down on my side—an ocean of bed between us. But little by little we edged toward the middle, until at last we were lying with our arms around each other.

I decided to ask if Cal could be excused from the research program. One of the doctors at the neurological center gave him the mini-mental test, which he had already had so many times. I sat beside him as he was being tested. He never complained. He tried his hardest. He couldn't answer any of the questions. When he was asked to draw a clock, he drew a straight line. The research team dismissed him.

One hard part of the whole experience was learning that the study done on the new drug was being stopped, as the results were unsatisfactory. Nobody seemed to know why the drug didn't work. I also learned later that people with Alzheimer's are no longer expected to stop their medications to enter a clinical trial, as this had been found to cause a sharp decline in some cases. I held on to the fact that for Cal being part of research to slow or even end the ravages of Alzheimer's had made him happy and given him the feeling that he could do something against the disease. I was proud of his willingness to volunteer for the study, and his courage. But for me, though I knew his decline was inevitable, it was unbearably sad that his efforts had been so costly.

Chapter Five

Things got progressively worse. As time went on, we were no longer alone. More and more invisible demons, or rather demons invisible to me, invaded our apartment. Cal could see and hear them clearly. He would warn me.

"Shhh. They're here. You'd better go away."

"Maybe if I put on a tape, they'll leave," I'd say.

"No, no. Just go. They want quiet."

When I explained this to Dr. Santulli, he said, "It's not uncommon for hallucinations to accompany Alzheimer's. We can put Cal back on some medications now, and I'll see if there's something I can increase a little. We can't stop the disease, but we can keep Cal from being frightened."

Cal remained confused. The only time he wasn't out of it was on the tennis court, where he still returned any ball hit to him effortlessly. One morning he couldn't remember how to take his pills. He'd swallow some water and then drop his pill in the water glass instead of in his mouth. We finally got through all his medications, but it took over half an hour.

Afterward I lay on our bed, exhausted. Out the window I watched a hawk circling without effort—up, down, around. "Take me with you," I wanted to cry out. "Let me ride on your wings. I'm tired of trying to fix mistakes, to make things work."

The Memory of All That

———

If Cal was doing poorly, clearly so was I. "Cal struggles with Alzheimer's," I wrote in my journal, "and I with weariness and sudden bouts of crying." One word of praise from anyone and tears began to cascade down my cheeks. During one of our office visits at Dartmouth Hitchcock with Dr. Santulli, he said, "You're handling all this very well, Mary."

I nodded thanks as the tears began. Dr. Santulli looked surprised. "What's this?" I hunched my shoulders to indicate I didn't know.

I left with a prescription for an anti-depressant, which surprised me. I had never thought of myself as depressed. The prescription was changed several times as I became allergic to whatever it was, until we finally found one that worked perfectly. I could now smile and say "thank you" if someone said something kindly or supportive. A relief. I now hardly ever cried, not even at the movies, which I actually sort of missed.

I also began seeing more of Ruth Whybrow, the social worker who led the Alzheimer's support group nearby. Calm and sympathetic, she was a great help. So was my garden. Friends had offered me bits from their plots—a small rose bush, some irises needing division. As summer began, Cal also seemed to be doing a bit better. He willingly came with me to the garden several days a week and dozed in a chair in the shade while I worked.

One morning at breakfast, looking over at him, I asked, "How're you feeling?"

"Amsterdam," he replied.

"Amsterdam?"

He nodded and smiled. "Yup. Amsterdam."

I smiled back. It seemed that Amsterdam was a pretty good feeling.

Cal was also able to walk along the river again for two miles each afternoon. Not that he always remembered what we did. One evening as we stood in line to check in for dinner, the woman in front of me turned and said, "Wasn't today beautiful?" I didn't recognize her or her husband, but she was obviously his caregiver. "We went down by the river, and it was so blue," she continued. "So was the sky, and the trees are so green. We had the nicest walk."

Cal was listening, and he turned to me and said, "Why don't we ever do that?" A year ago, I would have said, "We just did." Now, a little wiser, I touched his hand and replied, "Good idea. Maybe tomorrow."

Cal's oldest daughter, Joan, gave me a break, nicely offering to stay with her father for several days while I went up to the St. Lawrence River for a joint memorial service for my aunt and my cousin's husband. Mike, Cal's oldest son, had done a five-day stint earlier in the summer when I went to my grandson's high school graduation. I wrote out Cal's routine at length for her. "Don't try to plan any big projects," I cautioned at the end. "It's enough to make it through the day."

On my return, Joan said all had gone well. She clearly took very good care of Cal, evident in the detailed notes she left me. "Dad really loves to whistle to marching music," she concluded. Bless her.

Still, the doctors felt I was really worn out and needed at least four hours a day alone. It was true that I was tired. But I no longer felt comfortable leaving Cal by himself in the apartment.

The Memory of All That

I tried having a woman some of the other residents recommended, but Cal would have none of it. As soon as Nora entered our apartment and chirped, "And how are we today?" Cal rose from his chair, went into the bedroom, and closed the door.

Then I had a scare. Cal was in a real fog for several days. I waited through the weekend. We still played tennis but lost 6-0. By Monday I was so concerned I finally called the clinic, and one of the nurses came right up to see him. She found the plastic cup included with one of his medication refills had been marked wrong, with a red line drawn at 2.5 rather than .25 milligrams. I'd been giving Cal ten times the dosage he was supposed to get! Fortunately, it was only a mild tranquilizer and Cal recovered quickly, but I felt I had really let him down. I blamed myself for not having caught the mistake. One doctor had told me earlier that it was important for families to pay attention to the care of their loved ones, as small errors are common. The incident made me realize how very tired I was and that I needed more help with Cal.

Kendal did have some adult daycare, its Friendship Program. When we first arrived, there was no memory care unit. But patients with dementia were invited to come down to a special wing for several hours a day, from ten to two, with lunch included.

At first, I went with Cal to the program. He enjoyed the music and whistled along to all the songs, and the others loved to hear him do so. "He's the center of our program when he comes," the music director told me.

I had a lot of routine visits backed up—dentist, doctor, haircut. This would be a great solution, I thought. I could get some of these things taken care of and not worry, knowing Cal was in a safe place.

But how to explain my absence to Cal? His youngest daughter, Karen, always thoughtful and kind, called to say her friends, caring for parents with Alzheimer's, said just to tell him right before I left.

"Say you'll be back soon, you have an appointment, and that he'll have fun," she advised. "My friends say you can tell him the same thing every day and that you will both be happier."

"Thank you, Kare," I told her gratefully. "You make me feel less alone."

So I took Cal down to the Friendship Program and left him there on his own. Things went well. The nurses told me Cal only asked a few times when I would be back, and they showed him a card saying what time I would return.

"You were very late," Cal himself told me. But he wasn't angry or complaining.

The second visit went less well. I led Cal down to the Friendship Program, but he really didn't want me to leave. "Stay with me, please stay with me," he pleaded.

It was so hard to say no to him when he'd always done so much for me. But the doctors had told me to be firm. I took him to the nurse in charge, who tried to interest him in a puzzle. She urged me to go on to my dentist appointment, saying Cal would be fine. I went, but when I got back, Cal wasn't fine.

"He wouldn't stay," the nurse explained. "We tried everything, but he insisted on going back to your apartment. I finally let him go and sent an aide with him. They're up there now."

I ran up the steps rather than waiting for the elevator. The aide was sitting in a chair by our front door. Cal was pounding on the door, calling, "Let me in! Mary, let me in!"

I took his hand. "I'm here," I said. He grabbed me.

"Good" was all he said.

Later he began to talk. "Why are they sending me down there with all the worst people? Are they sending me down there to die?"

I kept trying to get Cal involved in the Friendship Program, but nothing worked. He consistently refused to take part in any of the activities, or even just stay in the room. The staff running the program simply could not afford to have an aide following Cal around every day. Finally, I was asked to a meeting of half a dozen people who had worked with Cal. They each briefly summarized their experiences with him, then told me that Cal was no longer welcome at their daily gathering. He had failed the Friendship Program.

"You've got to understand, Mary, Cal is what we call a 'Red,' the most difficult kind," I was told. "We just don't have the kind of help to give him what he needs."

I was angry. I also felt desperate. The Cal I loved was disappearing. I was losing him. I burst into tears. I, who couldn't stand to be seen crying, sat there sobbing while the whole group silently stared at me.

I told them that if they ever had more bad news, not to call a meeting to tell me, just to let me meet with the doctor alone. They apologized.

When I asked one of the nurses later what was meant by a "Red," she replied, "Someone who resists and fights the disease."

So now I took Cal with me everywhere, afraid to leave him alone even for a little while. I took him to the grocery store, the hairdresser when I got my hair cut, the dentist when I had my teeth cleaned, explaining beforehand that my husband had Alzheimer's and I couldn't leave him alone.

Once we went together to my eye doctor. I got Cal settled in a chair right across from me, and though eye contact was difficult with all the testing going on, I could murmur reassurances and measure how Cal was doing. Things went reasonably well for about fifteen minutes. Then Cal started taking off his shoes and socks. Wiggling his toes up and down, Cal demanded that Dr. Livingston, the eye doctor, examine his aching feet. Dr. Livingston's response was "Mary, I think that's enough for today. Call and we'll reschedule."

I knelt before Cal, put his shoes and socks back on, and acknowledged to myself that I needed to get more help. Nothing was working. Not medication, not the Friendship Program, not the "How are we today" caretaker.

"Dark times," I wrote in my journal that evening.

All our children had visited often since Cal and I had been at Kendal. Cal's younger two, Mark and Karen, spent a lot of time with us, and his two oldest children, Mike and Joan, had even stayed with him for a stretch. My daughters also came as much as they could, and my son Steve had flown several times all the way from Hawaii, where he lived, and called frequently. "How's Mom?" he'd ask, making me smile while enjoying his concern about me as well as Cal. But all of them were working very hard and lived far away.

Surely, there must be someone at the Dartmouth Medical School, I thought, who would understand Cal's tragic losses. Once a successful inventor with eighty patents, he now was not able to draw a clock or complete a sentence. Once a nationally ranked tennis and squash player, he now could not even throw the ball up to serve or make love anymore. How hard it must be for him, as well as me. I had to find the right person who could help us.

I wrote up a short description of Cal, stating the things he'd once done, that he had Alzheimer's, and that I would like to find a companion for him for a few hours a week. A nice woman at the medical school tacked the e-mail I'd written to a bulletin board, and to my surprise, I received seven replies from medical students interested in working with Cal.

Before I could answer them, the phone rang. It was a young woman named Carrie. Her boyfriend, a medical student, had brought home a copy of my letter, and she was calling because she wanted to apply for the job. "I'm aiming for medical school myself one of these days," she explained, "but right now I'm working here in the sleep center, and I have much more free time than my boyfriend does."

We arranged to meet in the lobby the next day.

Cal and I were already there when Kendal's front door opened, and sunshine and Carrie came in. She was smiling, blond curly hair tumbling over her shoulders, wearing a T-shirt, cutoffs, and sneakers.

I could tell Cal liked her right away from the way he stood and moved toward her.

We introduced ourselves, and I said to Cal, although really to Carrie, "I bet she'd like to see our pool and exercise room."

Cal seemed filled with more energy than I'd seen in weeks. He bounded along in front of us, and when we got to the exercise room, he showed off his strength by doing more on the Kaiser machines than Carrie could. She was properly admiring.

Up in our apartment I asked Carrie when she could start. "Tomorrow," she said.

I didn't know how to put it; others always stated their fee immediately. Awkwardly I asked, "How much do you charge?"

She looked surprised. "Nothing," she said. "I just want to do it."

My turn to be surprised. "No," I said, "we can't do it that way. Let me think about it, and I'll get back to you."

I thought and talked to Cal and ended up calling Carrie and telling her we'd love to have her with us, but it was important to us to pay what the "And how are we today?" woman had charged.

All through that summer and fall Carrie came two or three afternoons a week. Cal looked forward to her visits, and so did I. When I returned from my errands and appointments, I never quizzed them about what they had done. But one day, as I drove back to Kendal, I saw them walking side by side, Carrie's face turned up to Cal's, and I thought how happy and attractive they appeared.

Chapter Six

Carrie helped, as well as our friends, but the disease was getting worse; even I could see that. Evenings were hard. We no longer ate in the dining room. Cal found it difficult to wait for the waiter to bring our meals and would pound the table with his fists.

We switched to the café, which was much less formal than the main dining room, but this too was a challenge, as we had to take trays through a line and pick up our food. I tried to shuffle Cal in front of me while selecting a main course, salad, and something to drink for both of us.

In the old days Cal and I used to talk all the time, both of us saying what we thought, never trying to agree, switching from one topic to another, then switching back again, almost as though we were weaving something. When we went out to dinner, we used to look at couples eating in silence and say, "What's the matter with them? Why don't they talk to each other?" and then "We'll never be like that."

But that is exactly how we had become. Eating alone in the café, we were mostly silent. Cal rarely said anything. I would try to tell him small snippets of news, but he usually didn't respond.

Again, friends helped out. A wonderful couple who lived on

the floor above us suggested we eat dinner together each night. Cal was fond of both Edie and Charlie. Charlie somehow juggled Cal and two glasses of cranberry juice through the line and kept him happy while Edie and I picked up the rest of our food.

Cal would listen while we three talked and occasionally say something. One evening Edie asked me a question about Yelping Hill and Cal said, "Yelping Hill? Are we going to Yelping Hill?"

"Not this weekend, sweetie. Our good friends Marcia and Hal are coming to see us."

Cal looked at me. "Darn it," he said.

For some reason we all burst out laughing. Cal smiled, pleased that he'd said something we enjoyed.

As well as finding people to help us, I was learning to take other steps to make our life easier. We had never been big spenders, and our house in Englewood had had many of Cal's home-made inventions, like a burglar alarm of wires that snaked all across the ceiling of the basement and never really reassured me. Cal's old station wagon, which we used at Kendal, also had quirks and foibles. One day I told Cal, "We need a new car."

His youngest daughter, Karen, came to visit and offered to go with us to the auto dealership. While the salesman led me over to a model I liked, she tried to keep Cal busy. He was thrilled by the cars. He found a bright red one particularly fascinating and climbed in behind the steering wheel. As there was no key to turn, this seemed safe enough. But then it was time to leave. Cal had no intention of getting out of that car. Karen tried to coax him, then to gently pry his fingers off the steering wheel. Cal was not going to let go. Finally, I arrived. "Cal," I said, "come see the new car we're going to buy. I think you'll really like it." Intrigued, he finally left the driver's seat and followed me.

That car, though white, not red, was a pleasure for both of us. It took a week or so to finalize the sale, but the next time we went to the river, I drove us there in the new car. Cal loved it!

All through our marriage, long before Alzheimer's appeared, Cal had supported me, taking my side no matter what. When we were still living in Englewood, I had been in a minor automobile accident in Tenafly, the adjacent town. A bus and I collided; actually, I was waiting for the bus to pass when instead it rammed into me. The driver got out and yelled at me for running into him. A passenger leaned out of his window and shouted, "Don't listen to him. He's done this before."

I was upset. But when I started to tell Cal about it that evening, he said, "Sweetheart, forget about it. Just know whatever happens, whether you're right or wrong, I'm on your side. Okay?"

I was stunned. Nobody had ever said anything like that to me before. I treasured his words. I still do. I knew my parents had supported me, but I also felt I had to earn their support, deserve it, and prove myself, and I tried very hard to do so. Cal, though, seemed to believe that with love came automatic support. I wanted to become that kind of person. Over the years, Cal's statement, "I'm on your side," had helped me through many rough spots.

Late one day at Kendal, as the fall progressed, Cal unexpectedly soiled himself. Naked, he ran from the apartment down the hall. When I realized what had happened, I grabbed a quilt from our bed and ran after him. I caught up with him when he tumbled down on the floor, covering his face with his hands. "I made a mess," he said. I knelt beside him and wrapped the quilt around him and whispered, "Sweetheart, forget about it. Whatever happens, I'm on your side. You know that."

Little by little he took his hands down and looked at me, and then gave me a small shaky kind of smile. I could almost hear him saying, "Copycat."

But all of this was very hard on Cal. One night before we slept, Cal, who was usually asleep before I was, tossed and turned and then muttered, "I want to die."

Chilled, I exclaimed, "Oh, sweetheart, please don't say that. I would miss you so much." It was true—I would miss him. Despite the daily frustrations and work—the endless questions—the lack of any time alone. There would never be anyone like him.

In the morning, lying close to him, wanting to hold on to him, I whispered, "Maybe you meant sleep?"

"Maybe," he mumbled.

Later, I wished I'd been less selfish, more courageous, and let him talk more about what he really wanted.

That November 1998, Cal's daughters came to visit again, to celebrate his seventy-ninth birthday—Joan from Maine and Karen from Florida. I was so glad to have them with us.

The first afternoon, while Cal was out for a walk with our friends Betsy and Sandy, his daughters and I went to see Dr. Santulli for a long talk. He suggested that perhaps it was time for Cal to move down to Whittier, a new section of the Health Center recently set up for those with advanced dementia. It was in the same place where the Friendship Program had once been held. I remembered how Cal had felt about that program. His words rang clearly in my head: "Why are they sending me to the place where all the worst people are? Are they sending me down there to die?" How would he ever agree to go there permanently? How could I ever let him go there? But Carrie had said she would continue to come, and that would help. Maybe between us we could make it work.

Karen spoke up, asking, "How will it be for Mary? I know it's probably best for Dad, but I want to be sure it's all right for Mary too."

Dr. Santulli said, "I think it's right for her as well, although she can tell us if I'm wrong about that. But Mary is very worn out, more than she lets on."

"Is there an empty room?" Joan asked.

"There is," said Dr. Santulli, "all furnished and ready."

"Good," said Joan. "I've brought a few things to make it homey, some pillows I embroidered, pictures, things like that." I realized Joan and Karen had probably been talking to each other about such a move.

"Okay," Dr. Santulli responded, "I'll call down to Doris, the head nurse, and let her know you're coming."

Dr. Santulli guided us toward Whittier, the Alzheimer's wing, introduced us to Doris, the head nurse, and showed us the room that would be Cal's. It was a nice room with windows looking out on a garden, a high hospital bed, a bureau and a chair, and a small bathroom.

"You can bring anything else you'd like to make it more familiar for Cal," Doris said. "Maintenance will help you."

Dr. Santulli then handed me three packets of pills, two marked *Cal*, the other *Mary*. "Directions are inside. You take yours tonight, Mary. Give Cal the pink ones tonight and the white ones at breakfast. These will help you both sleep and keep Cal calm in the morning. You can also pick up a wheelchair to bring him down, if you wish."

Joan, Karen, and I went to work arranging Cal's room. I knew Cal was still with Betsy and Sandy. Soon, though, I had to leave. I couldn't stay any longer. It was just too hard to think of Cal being down in this room all alone.

But when I got back to the apartment, I called maintenance and had them take Cal's favorite lounge chair and the wooden card table we'd bought in our first days at Kendal down to the room in Whittier. I sent a quilt he had always liked. Then I made myself return. Joan and Karen were busy decorating the walls of his room with pictures of the family. Joan showed me the pillows she had covered in navy-blue with red trim and carefully embroidered with the letters of Cal's name. Karen gave me a quick hug.

Cal was in our apartment when we got back upstairs. Betsy and Sandy left, and Cal settled down to opening his birthday presents. His daughters knelt beside him, helping him untie ribbons and read the birthday cards.

"Happy birthday, dear Dad. Happy birthday to you!" Joan and Karen sang

I can't remember what the presents were, but I did take several pictures, and in them Cal is smiling, his daughters on either side of him, though his eyes look dark and sunken.

Nor can I remember what we had for dinner. I do remember getting Cal ready for bed—helping him into his pajamas, helping him wash, grinding up the pink pills and mixing them with some cinnamon applesauce, lying down beside him till I thought he was asleep.

After a few minutes I joined Karen and Joan in the living room, and then the three of us moved to the den so our talk wouldn't wake Cal.

But shortly Cal was standing in the doorway of the den, looking at us. I was up immediately. "Hi, darling," I said. "Can I get you something?"

Cal put his arms around me. "I just want to be with my girls."

He settled on the couch and gathered us around him. We stayed like that for almost an hour, reminiscing, laughing, all of us glad to be together. The girls, I learned later, stayed up all night talking.

When Cal fell asleep on the couch, Joan and Karen half-carried him back to bed. Later I lay awake beside him, remembering the past, memorizing Cal. I had purposely not taken the pills Dr. Santulli had given me. Would this be the last time we would lie together?

I took off Cal's old T-shirt that I always slept in these days and fit my naked body against his blue pajamas. I matched my breathing to his but moved back a little so my tears would soak my pillowcase, not Cal's pajamas.

The next morning Cal was groggy but compliant. He let me dress him and lead him out to the breakfast table. His daughters quickly surrounded him. I poured Cal's orange juice, and while he drank it, I mixed the last of Dr. Santulli's potions with strawberry jam and spread it on his toast. Almost immediately after he'd finished it, his eyes began to close, and his head lolled to one side.

"He's asleep," Joan whispered. "I'll be right back."

I sat close to Cal, worried that he might slip from his chair. Karen sat tight beside me. Neither of us spoke.

Joan came in pushing a wheelchair. "Yesterday Dr. Santulli said we might need this."

All three of us worked to slide Cal from his chair at the table into the wheelchair. Joan fastened a strap across her father's chest, and Karen held the door to the apartment open while Joan pushed Cal through it.

When they'd gone, Karen and I put our arms around each

other. "Judas," I whispered. "I feel like a traitor. I shouldn't have let him go."

Karen hugged me. "It was time," she said, "and he won't be far away."

She was right. That was why Cal and I had come to Kendal, so we could still be together under the same roof, even when his disease grew too much for him to stay with me.

Part IV

WHITTIER

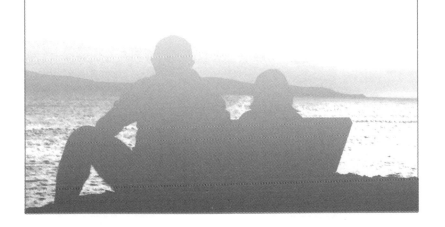

November 1998

Nov. 17th

I wake to an empty bed—no one beside me. My life has shrunk to a sharp focus on the immediate present. I can't think beyond that.

The whole apartment seems eerily quiet. Where are the girls?

As if on cue they come in. Joan says, "We've been down to say goodbye to Dad. He's still asleep, but please tell him we went to see him before we left."

They pack quickly, kiss me goodbye, and soon are on their way home.

I hold back the tears until they are gone, but then the tears become sobs. I go to the bathroom and turn on the water to cover the noise. Why had I let the doctors, the nurses, the family talk me into letting Cal be moved to the memory care unit? He won't understand where he is when he wakes up. Guilt sours my stomach.

Finally, I wipe away the tears. What good are they? My thoughts center on Cal in Whittier. Is he all right? Is he still asleep? I checked last night, and the nurse said he roused around five in the evening and had some tea and toast. But did he sleep the whole night through after that? If not, who was with him?

I know the head nurse told me it would be best if I stayed away for a few days to let Cal get "acclimated," but I worry he'll be frightened when Dr. Santulli's sleep potion wears off and he finds himself in a strange place.

I pull on my red warm-up suit and go downstairs quickly—walking as fast as I can, not running, not wanting to call attention to myself. Suppose someone stops me and wants to know where I'm going? If I say Whittier, they might tell me it's too soon. I'm not supposed to go yet, but I can't hold myself back.

Now I'm almost there. The halls are empty. Cal's door is closed. Quietly, quietly I approach the door and slowly, gradually, I open it.

And there he is, lying on his right side, as always. *Please, God*, I pray, not even sure what I'm asking for. Cal opens his eyes. I kneel beside the bed so we'll be on the same level and touch his face.

"There you are," he says.

"Yes," I reply, smiling at his familiar words. But now I hear voices down the hall. "Do you need anything?" I ask.

Cal moves his head a little, which I take to be a "no."

"I'll be back," I promise.

I find Doris, the head nurse, in her office. She raises her eyebrows, and before she can speak, I say, "I came to see what you need for Cal. I suddenly realized that when his daughter brought him down yesterday, we didn't send anything with him—not even a toothbrush."

"Well—we could use some clothes for him."

A long pause.

Then Doris says, "All right. Bring them here to me."

I smile and go back to Cal, who is raised up on one elbow. I kiss him and say, "I won't be long. I'm going to get you some clean clothes."

A half hour later I return with a duffel bag of slacks, shirts and shoes, underwear, socks, pajamas, a couple of sweaters, and his shaving kit and toothbrush.

Both his room and his bed are empty. I leave the bag and go looking for Cal.

I find him at a little table eating shredded wheat and bananas.

Doris appears, and I quickly say, "I put the bag with his clothes and toiletries in his room. How are things going?"

Doris smiles for the first time. "Fine," she says. "Cal hasn't given us a bit of trouble."

I smile in return. I want to have a good relationship with her, though I don't intend to cower.

I sit down for a moment and survey the surroundings. Whittier is obviously a make-do of what was once another part of the hospital wing. Here in an open area are four or five small tables and chairs set up as an improvised dining room. The wide hallway beyond is arranged as a sort of living room.

There is a tiny room at the other end of the hall that seems to be the kitchen. I have already been in Doris's office. Farther down the hall, past Cal's room, are a few more doors—some open, some closed—which I assume belong to other patients.

"How many others are here?" I ask.

"We have eight patients overall, counting Cal. They'll be out in a little while. We're getting everyone cleaned up now."

"A busy place," I reply and rise, hug Cal's shoulder, and say, "See you later," to both of them.

I go back to our apartment and shower and dress. I need to get organized, plan how to live this new kind of life. I decide that there will be no hard-and-fast rules. We'll just sort of let it work itself out. The most important thing will be to spend time with Cal. I'll try to go down each day at midmorning and midafternoon. I'll take down some cards and some music, and maybe we can walk a little.

Nov. 18th

When I go down this morning, Doris tells me Cal has had a good night, though he was late waking and didn't eat much of the breakfast she took him. But he seemed in a good mood. "He gave me a smile," she says.

In the afternoon I find Cal sitting in a wheelchair eating lunch. Doris explains that since he wouldn't come out of his room any other way, they brought him out in his chair. "He should be with the others," she says. I agree.

Cal is willing to walk with me a bit after he finishes his lunch. "Be quick," he says, though.

Nov. 19th

Doris says Cal was upset this morning before I arrived, swinging his arms around and holding her hand too hard. He eventually settled down.

I pull up a chair beside Cal. He grabs both my hands, squeezing them, more in fear, it seems, than a gesture of affection.

When I arrive in the afternoon, Cal seems better, alert, talkative. Dr. Santulli has been to check on him and adjust his medications. Cal is in the living room and willing to stay there. He doesn't mind when I leave to do laundry for him.

Nov. 21st

By the end of the week, we are into a loose routine. I go down at ten or ten thirty in the morning. Usually most of the people whose names I'm learning are gathered in the music room. There's Howard, a doctor; Nancy and Jane, both former teachers; and Margaret, who paints; Willie, a grocery store manager;

and Holly and Phyllis, who I don't know yet. The music room, which I assume was once a patient's room, now contains a piano and eight or ten chairs. Crowded.

Most mornings Cal is still in his room when I get there, usually dressed and maybe shaved, lying on his bed. He sits up and smiles when he sees me.

I say, "Good morning, darling," and he raises his face for a kiss. "I love you," I say.

"I love you too," he replies.

This is our morning ritual, the same each day.

December 1998

Dec. 2nd

This morning when I arrive, I encourage Cal to get up. I worry that he will lose strength in his legs, and I know how he would hate to be confined to a wheelchair. He wriggles off the bed. I take his hand and lead him to the music room.

Today, Janet, a volunteer, is playing the piano and singing along with a couple of the nurses and a few of the patients. The feeling in the room is friendly. No one seems to be required to do anything—encouraged but not required.

We find two chairs together. The voices rise: "She'll be comin' round the mountain when she comes." I join in softly. My ability to carry a tune isn't that great, but I sing. When the music starts again, I whisper to Cal, "Why don't you whistle?" and a few bars into "I've Been Workin' On the Railroad," Cal does begin to whistle, right on tune, and everybody loves it.

Dec. 7th

In our next visits to the music room, Cal continues to whistle when the others sing, and he claps along with them when the song is done. It's nice to see him enjoying himself, and it's important for me to have happy moments to hold on to.

Dec. 9th

Cal is loving with me. He lets me shave him. He walks beside me in the halls of Kendal. Often, he doesn't want to, but I urge him on. So we continue, sometimes in very tiny steps—the effect of medication, I am told. It isn't easy to see him walk like this, he who not so long ago had run swiftly around squash and tennis courts and danced gracefully across polished floors. But it's nice that he still wants to hold my hand.

Dec. 15th

This morning Doris tells me Cal ate a huge breakfast of French toast. Then she adds, "He eloped last night." Apparently, he got up in the middle of the night and left Whittier, heading down the hall toward the rest of Kendal, but one of the staff soon found him and brought him back. "We're going to give him a 'wandering bracelet,'" Doris explains. Apparently, this will set off an alarm if Cal tries to leave Whittier again.

When I come down for my afternoon visit, I find Cal asleep on the living room floor. I wake him, and we sit side by side holding hands for a bit, listening to Christmas carols playing on the radio. Cal smiles at me.

"How much do you love me?" I ask.

"One hundred percent," he answers.

Dec. 25th

My daughter Susan visits for Christmas. Sometimes Cal seems to know her, other times not. All our other children call on Christmas Day. We open the presents they have sent. He has fun ripping off the bright wrapping paper and seeing what's inside each package. I always feel lighter when Cal is happy.

January 1999

Jan. 4th

Just before I left this morning, Cal said, "They've caught me with too many drugs."

"Too many drugs?" I asked

"Yes," he said, and then fell back on his pillow.

Jan. 7th

Our resident doctor has taken a leave for a bit, but her replacement, a short, balding, cheerful man, Dr. Wilson, comes to see how Cal is doing. He seems quite competent, and he makes Cal smile. Dr. Santulli also visits again and says he will decrease some of Cal's medications.

Jan. 11th

Cal is now completely off one of the drugs used to keep him calm during the move to Whittier. This afternoon when I arrive, I find him on his bed, very upset, trembling all over. Apparently, one of the aides had to help him in the bathroom, and this distressed him. He is trying to take his clothes off. "We have to get out of here," he tells me.

Another aide comes in and calms him down. He eats every bit of his dinner after I leave, I'm told later, and a big bowl of ice cream—happy.

Jan. 14th

Cal's days are mixed. Some are good, some not so good. I go down to see him every morning. It is always the same; he is lying on his bed. The nurses say he comes to all his meals, but other than that, he rarely leaves his room or his bed. He never gives them any trouble except during times of dressing and toileting. How hard that must be for him, a proud and private man.

Along with his favorite chair, I had a radio, magazines, and a book or two put in his room, and his daughters did a wonderful job filling it with cheerful cushions and family pictures,. But Cal seems totally unaware of any of it. He is almost always dressed when I arrive but often unshaved. The nurses say sometimes he won't let them near him. His nurses and aides are a wonderful bunch, though; they remain kind, patient, and pleasant.

Jan. 16th

I worry, not a usual thing for me. I hate to think of Cal alone in his room lying on top of his bed. What can I do? The question gnaws at me. I wake up in the middle of the night and think, *I know, I'll take down a tennis ball*. Why I think this will help I'm not sure, but the next day I tuck a yellow tennis ball into the basket of clean clothes. I leave it there all morning, not sure what to do with it. It seems out of place in Whittier, but in the afternoon I get it out and bounce it a few times.

Cal is watching me, and out of the blue I say, "Let's play catch."

Surprisingly, Cal doesn't object, and we stand between the bed and the dresser and bounce the ball back and forth between us. But there isn't enough room, and when I miss the ball, it rolls under the bed or some equally awkward place. "We need more space," I say and head for the hall.

Cal follows me silently. We stand almost twelve feet apart and again bounce the ball to each other. Cal's eye-hand coordination is still good; mine is still poor. He catches the ball easily, sometimes with his right hand, sometimes with his left, no matter how off my throw is.

We've been in the hall about ten minutes when one of the nurses stops in front of me and catches the ball and throws it back to Cal. Now there are three of us playing. Another nurse joins us, then an aide. Now we are five. Cal is having fun. He fakes a throw to one of us and then tosses it to somebody else. He throws it from behind his back or between his legs, and pretty soon we are all laughing.

Jan. 20th

The nurses tell me that ever since playing catch in the hall, Cal comes out of his room willingly. He never relates to the other patients, but he does to the nurses. They tell me that in the evening when everyone else is in bed, Cal appears and sits in the hall with them, and they share whatever snack they are having. During the day they find little chores for him to do, like putting the clean silverware away. He loves being useful. I am very grateful.

February 1999

Feb. 5th

This morning I went to see Ruth Whybrow, the social worker who led our Alzheimer's group up here near Kendal. I'd also begun to see her one-on-one when Cal worsened. It is always both comforting and useful to talk to her. I told her that for the first time in many months Cal seems happier, and that this is such a relief. I even feel I can take little trips away, leaving him in safe hands.

Feb. 10th

I went to Cal's "care plan" meeting this morning, where several of the doctors, nurses, and aides interacting with Cal are present. Everyone there said he is doing much better than before he moved down to Whittier and since his first weeks in the unit. The staff feel they have learned how to best relate to Cal. Only one or two interact with him at a time, no more, always speaking quietly. He is out in the living room and music room more often, is more talkative, and smiles frequently.

I go to see Cal after dinner. He is still in the dining room, dozing in a chair. He wakes briefly, says, "Hello, darling," and then goes back to sleep.

The Memory of All That

Feb. 15th

I went away for the first time since Cal's been in Whittier, driving over to Vermont a few days ago to ski with some of his old
Princeton classmates. It was fun planning the trip, and driving,
and seeing old friends. I only stayed overnight, though, leaving
early the next morning, as the weather report was bad.

Back at Kendal, I rushed down at once to see Cal, before
even unpacking. He was more interested in his fifth helping of
sweet potatoes than seeing me. I was slightly hurt but mainly
relieved. It makes me feel as though a heavy weight has been
lifted off me when he's content.

Feb. 17th

Carrie, the pretty young companion I found for Cal, has continued to visit him in Whittier. But today she comes up to my
apartment to see me after spending time with Cal. She says he
has had a good afternoon. She herself is sick again, though, with
a bad cough. She tells me she will come three more times to
help Cal adjust but then has to stop seeing him. She still cares
about him, but she is too overworked.

Feb. 27th

Carrie sends me a note saying she has loved being with Cal but
feels that he is at a stage now where he needs more experienced
care. I accept this and write telling her how much I appreciate
the happiness she'd given Cal and enclose her final check.

So now it is pretty much Cal and me and the Whittier
staff, and it makes me realize how much I miss our family. It is
nobody's fault. We picked Kendal at Hanover for two reasons:
it seemed like the best and kindest place for Cal, and the town

was familiar to him, as he had helped install one of his inventions, off-peak air conditioning, in the big hospital in Hanover.

I still think Kendal is the right place, but it is far from family. All Cal's four children have visited many times. It has been very hard for them to see their father so diminished, but they are very loving with him. My children have visited also. Still, I wish so that at least some of them, one or two of them, lived nearby.

Feb. 28th

I've decided that since this is where Cal will be from now on that I would like to get to know the people here better.

The memory care unit is very new, only four months old, and everyone is still learning. Just yesterday, the dining room became the living room and the living room the dining room. Everyone agrees it works better this way, at least so far. Besides these and the kitchen and the music room, there is also an office, a shower room, a tub room, several small rooms for medicine and such, and eleven bedrooms, each with a small bathroom with a sink and toilet.

Eventually, Whittier will be totally redone. There will be a large sunny dining room, an efficient kitchen, a TV room, a laundry room, and an attractive living room, as well as fourteen private rooms. But during our time it is rather bare and crowded. There isn't even a washing machine. I carry Cal's dirty clothes up to the laundry room on our third floor each night, wash and dry them, and take them back downstairs the next morning. If some things are lacking, though, kindness and thoughtfulness are plentiful.

There are three shifts of nurses: 7 p.m. to 3 a.m., 3 a.m. to 11 a.m., and 11 a.m. to 7 p.m. On each shift there is a registered nurse and two certified nursing assistants, an exceptional amount of support. All of the nurses and aides are kind and dedicated. Cal has been here over three months now, and I have yet to hear any of them say a cross word.

There are eight full-time residents and a few others who come during the day occasionally. The first room on the right belongs to Howard, the former dean of a good medical school. He is tall, distinguished, with a full head of white hair. He needs a walker now, otherwise he's apt to fall, and for much of the day he pushes the walker up and down the hall. He talks a great deal and is very genteel, always saying please and thank you. He often talks of having written books that don't exist and insists his wife is going to divorce him, though she has no intention of doing so and comes each day to visit. I've been told he ran a very tight ship when he was dean. Now he's quite sweet. We all smile when the phone rings in the living room and he picks up the leaf of a nearby plant and announces, "Good morning, Howard Woodson here." When he gets agitated occasionally, the nurses sit him down with a pad of paper and a pencil, and he calms at once, making notes of some kind.

Next to Howard's room is Nancy's. I barely know her. She's a sweet-faced, white-haired, fine-looking woman who is almost always in her room, usually under the covers of her bed.

Across the hall from Cal is Jane. Jane has a thick head of gray hair and is always well-dressed. She often walks the hall, singing, right on key, a Christmas carol or a ballad. Most times she carries "Kitty," a large stuffed animal, which is very real to her. She is very protective of "Kitty." She also gives advice from time to time. Last Wednesday, Cal and I were also walking in the hall, Cal moving slowly because of his latest prescription, an anti-psychotic drug he'd been given to allay some of his imagined fears. Unfortunately, the side effects produce symptoms similar to Parkinson's disease—trembling, a shuffling walk, and rigidity. Halfway down the hall Jane confronted us. "Oh, that man doesn't treat you right," she said to me. "You give him hell when you get him home."

Holly's room is close to Jane's. Holly's hair is dark, streaked with gray, and her smile comes easily. She is usually quiet but always sings when Ellen, the music therapist, plays the piano or guitar. Holly knows all the words to the "old-time songs"— Stephen Foster, hymns, "Yankee Doodle," "She'll Be Coming Round the Mountain," and many more. I don't know Holly very well. She is sometimes in a wheelchair, but so far I haven't seen any indications of Alzheimer's, though she must have some kind of dementia or she wouldn't be in the unit.

On the other side of the hall is Willie, big, rangy, and strong. A black cap usually covers his thinning hair. Willie asks questions and sometimes talks to himself. I can't understand him, but the nurses can. They kid around with Willie and are very sweet with him. Willie is the former head of the produce section of a large supermarket. His favorite occupation now is moving furniture; most often he moves chairs from one end of the hall to the other. Last Friday, he brought a typewriter down to the living room. One of the nurses on the morning shift thanked him and then took it back to where it had come from.

Then there's Cal, the only person new to the group, and probably the youngest, at least the youngest looking, still trim with dark hair, and when he smiles, handsome.

At the end of the hall Margaret and Phyllis have rooms next to each other. Margaret is small and quiet. The nurses tell me that Margaret never spoke before she came to Whittier, when the unit opened in August. She still doesn't say much, but she answers questions, sings, and smiles. Phyllis's husband, Bud, who's a doctor, says, "Phyllis is a different woman now, much happier, since the unit opened up. Margaret too."

Whittier also has some day patients. The only one I've met is Ruthie. She lives in the regular unit of the main hospital in Kendal. Her family visits her often and is loving with her, but I've never seen any of them down in Whittier. They may not come to our unit, but Ruthie does. Little and quick, she dances through the plaid curtain that serves as the door to Whittier during the daylight hours. Usually, she is without shoes and full of smiles, almost joyous despite her failing mind. The nurses all love her and put their arms around her when she visits, which is almost every day, and dance with her if there's music playing. It is difficult to believe she's had Alzheimer's for seven years. When Ruthie gets tired, she finds a corner in a quiet place, tucks her arms under her head, and sleeps.

But not everyone loves Ruthie. Before the Whittier unit was opened, the patients with dementia were scattered throughout the three other health-care units. Many of them wandered, Ruthie among them, not only up and down the halls but in and out of other patients' rooms, occasionally taking something that appealed to them. Some of the other patients were just back from surgery and still connected to various life-support systems. They were both frightened and angered by the invasion of, to them, the "scary people."

Patients with dementia sometimes also wandered outside Kendal as well, and this was worrisome because a busy highway runs right past our entrance. Once, during a dark, cold night, Ruthie had to be brought back from a gully by the town police. And the last time, she was found on Main Street, three miles from our retirement home.

Because of these incidents, Ruthie and others were given "wandering bracelets," locks and alarms were put on doors, and our memory care unit, Whittier, was set up. Now secure in their own place, Whittier's residents rarely stray. They seem to feel comfortable and safe here. Even Cal, who refused to stay for just a few hours in the Friendship Program, climbing three flights of stairs to pound on our apartment door, and who tried to go off on his own one of his first nights here, now must be coaxed to go with me for a walk outside the unit.

I hope that when my time comes, I will be in as safe and loving a place as Whittier.

March 1999

Mar. 1st

We are all worried about Bud, Phyllis's husband. Evidently, his arteries are terribly clogged, and his heart is in such bad shape that an operation isn't possible. He told me the other day he only hopes he can last as long as his wife, Phyllis, does. They are very devoted. Bud still lives in their apartment but comes down daily for two or three lengthy visits, and Phyllis's face lights up when he enters the room. He is looking increasingly frail to me, though.

    Phyllis herself is tall, a little taller than Bud, and spare, with strong cheekbones. She seldom complains and had seemed to me to be more rooted in reality than most of the others. Then she asked me to walk with her the other day when Cal was sleeping, or pretending to be asleep. She said she liked the colors of my sweater and took my hand. We started down the hall, which was empty, and I told her how lucky she was to have such a nice husband. She stopped, looked directly at me, and said, "Oh, we're not married yet." I knew they had been married twenty-five years or more.

Mary MacCracken

Mar. 7th

I come down to find Cal sitting on his bed, dressed but with only socks on his feet. I put his shoes on and urge him to get up and either go for a walk or join the others who are singing in the music room. Cal heads for the music room, and Ellen, the music therapist, who is at the piano, welcomes us. From what she says, I gather that she tried to persuade him to come earlier but didn't get anywhere. Once there, Cal enjoys himself, whistling on tune with every song that is played, as well as whistling solo without piano accompaniment.

A couple of times a week, a few children from the day care center we have here at Kendal come to visit Whittier, and five or six are here today. Unlike many adults, the children aren't frightened by Alzheimer's, and they love hearing Cal whistle. They gather around him and try to whistle too. Before they go back to their playroom, they shake hands with each adult and say goodbye.

Mar. 15th

Bud, Phyllis's husband, had a heart attack in a Hanover pharmacy yesterday morning. My neighbors, who chanced to be in town, saw him carried into an ambulance and driven off to Dartmouth Hitchcock Medical Center. The nurses in Whittier say Bud is resting and will be back in a few days. No one has said anything to Phyllis.

Mar. 18th

It's a sad time in the memory care unit. Bud died in the hospital around four yesterday morning. His children are all here, staying in their parents' apartment, but he had instructed the nurses not to wake them if he should die in the night, typical of his thoughtfulness. Today, the children told their mother that Bud was gone. They said she shed a few tears and then went to sleep.

Sleep is the way many Alzheimer's patients deal with their disease. I know Cal closes his eyes whenever something comes up that he doesn't want to hear or do, like taking medicine or brushing his teeth. He also does fall into a deep snoring sleep a great deal. But whether this is due to medication or a desire to escape is hard to tell.

And now today Ruthie died. No more smiles and dancing, but most of us feel both sad and glad. Sad about missing Ruthie but glad that she went quickly, painlessly, from a silent heart attack.

Mar. 24th

The gathering room was full this past Sunday for Bud's memorial service. His children and friends spoke of his kindness, his devotion to Phyllis, and their love of a summer camp where he had been the director and doctor for many years. The service closed with the camp's hymn.

Ruthie's service was the following day. I see now why people like to take vacations from Kendal—too many deaths and too many memorials. But we have come here in part for care as we approach the end of our lives, and I have to remind myself that I have always believed that "to everything there is a season . . . a time to be born and a time to die."

The memorial, a Quaker one, was lovely. I had never been to one before. There was no music, hymns, bible reading, or praying, only silence until someone felt moved to speak. The first twenty minutes no one said anything; then from the far side of the room, a woman in her mid-fifties, dressed in a green uniform, stood up and said, "I clean the Sturges' apartment. I've known Ruthie for seven years, and I've never seen a sweeter smile than hers."

I found the service moving, drawn again to the Quakers' belief that everyone is equal. I decided during the silences that I would write another book, as Cal has wanted, about Alzheimer's. It seems something I may be able to give to others.

April 1999

Apr. 5th

Life goes on much the same in Whittier, despite our sad losses.
I come down this morning, and Cal and I go into the living
room where a nurse is doing proverbs with Holly, Willie, Margaret, and Phyllis. The nurse reads, "A penny saved is a . . .?"
Willie dozes. Phyllis rolls up the edge of her skirt and talks to
herself.

Margaret and Holly complete almost all the proverbs. Cal
occasionally picks up on a specific word—repeats it, adds to
it—but without any relation to the proverb. His eyes are open;
he looks interested. After about twenty minutes he stands up
and walks out. I follow. I am always glad when Cal is willing to
walk.

Today he walks well. We go out past the curtain that marks
the entrance and exit to Whittier. Cal now wears his "wandering bracelet" that will set off alarms. Small unobtrusive devices
placed at the curtain and at intervals along the walls signal care-
takers if a patient is out of any of the health-care units. Moving
ahead of Cal, I turn the alarms off as I have been shown to do.
I thought the bracelet would bother Cal. Many of the patients
regularly cut them off. But Cal doesn't seem to mind it. I think
he thinks of his bracelet as his watch.

We walk down to the exercise room. I always hope Cal will want to go in for a few minutes, but he never does now. We look at the pictures on the hall walls, pick up a local paper from our mailbox, and then Cal leads the way outdoors.

Months before, in the fall when Cal was rebelling and fighting against the disease as hard as he could, this might have been alarming, although even then he never tried to run away outside. Now his steps are small, and I am almost as strong as he is.

We walk outside for five or ten minutes and then head back for lunch.

In the afternoon we go for a drive along the river. Cal still loves my new car. Our friends Betsy and Sandy come with us. We all walk a bit, and then Cal and I wait in the car, listening to music, while they go a bit farther on and come back.

Apr. 9th

I decide to go over Cal's medications again with the nurses. I think one of them he gets four times a day may be the reason he slumps so much when he's sitting. On the other hand, it may make him easier for the staff to handle.

Apr. 12th

I am writing in bed this morning when the phone rings and Cal's new doctor, Dr. Wilson, says, "Mary, I'm calling because I heard from one of the nurses that you questioned the increase of one of the medications that I ordered. I think you need to understand that Cal has a terminal disease, and the best we can do for him is to try and make him comfortable and keep him from disturbing other people."

I say nothing. Then, "Thank you." I can't talk anymore and hang up.

I sit on the edge of my bed, my hand still on the phone. Why did I thank him—for what? Why did it hurt? I already knew everything he said. I guess it was the word *terminal*. I know, of course, that Cal isn't going to get better. I have learned that Alzheimer's doesn't reverse itself—but even though it's true, no one until now has used that word *terminal*. The word pounds inside my head—*TERMINAL*—*terminal*—*TERMINAL*.

Dear God, how much longer do we have?

Apr. 22nd

Actually, as the week passes, I am grateful for the doctor's call, because his words remind me that the time Cal and I have together is limited, and I want to fill Cal's days, our days, with as much joy as I can.

Blessedly, the weather has turned lovely. Clean air, bright sun, and the kind of blue sky I've seen only in New Hampshire.

"Come on, Cal," I say. "It's absolutely wonderful outside. Let's go for a ride."

"Okay."

Cal maneuvers himself into the front seat, not an easy task. I keep my hand on the top of his head so he won't bump it. Slowly he moves first one foot and then the other, then slides himself across the leather seat. I lean in the door and reach across him and fasten his seatbelt. I take a moment as I cross to the driver's seat to toss up another thank-you, because I'm not sure how much longer Cal will be able to get himself into the car. I love having him beside me. I fasten my own seatbelt, and we're off.

We drive to our favorite spot and park on River Road. I switch on the tape, and we listen to Ella Fitzgerald's songs, the songs we used to dance to. No more dancing now, but we hold hands.

Cal's eyes are bright today, and he's aware of everything around him. He comments on a speedboat and the water skier, the police car that passes us, lights flashing.

"Wonder where he's going," Cal says.

"Want to follow him?" I inquire.

Cal shakes his head. "I like it here."

"Me too," I say.

We stay for almost an hour. I leave the tape on during the drive back, and Ella sings, "I got rhythm—I got music—I got my man—Who could ask for anything more?"

I sing along. Crazy as it sounds, two old people, one terminally ill, are together and happy. Who could ask for anything more?

May 1999

May 10th

Cal is still very much aware, but it's difficult for him to find the right words for what he wants to say. This has been true from the beginning of Alzheimer's but is increasing now. His biggest loss throughout this disease has been language. It's extremely hard for him to communicate verbally. This loss is painful for both of us.

He does seem to have an ample supply of swear words, though, most of which I have never heard before, at least not from him. The nurse I talk to about this understands, as long as he swears quietly and doesn't disturb the other patients. She says, "It's the only way he can express anger at what's happening to him."

Lunch is served at twelve. I pour his milk, butter his potato, and cut anything that needs cutting, and when Cal becomes utterly involved with eating, I leave. I am back at two thirty. We go for our drive up River Road. Today we walk a little bit, then sit by the water with the car door open and hold hands and listen to our old familiar songs:

Mary MacCracken

"The way you hold your knife
The way you sing off key
The way you changed my life
No, no, they can't take that away from me."

Then back to dinner for both of us, and the day is done.

May 20th

Yesterday, I was struggling and unfortunately was not very good at Cal's "care planning" or "progress" meeting, which I am supposed to attend with some of the staff members at Kendal every three months or so. Each reported on their latest interactions with Cal. About halfway through, tears began to sneak out of my eyes. People, about half a dozen around a large table, began to push a Kleenex box toward me. I finally had to say, "Excuse me."

I got up, got a glass of water, and at last was able to go back and tell them how strange people are frightening to Cal; that intimate, invasive procedures are very difficult; that Cal's swearing is not "verbally abusive" but, as one of the nurses has explained, the only words he has for fear and frustration. I also explained his need for physical therapy, and my wish for a washing machine and dryer in Whittier. So it wasn't a total disaster. But it was hard to sit there and hear them read out things like "completely unable to dress himself," "totally unable to bathe," on and on. It felt like the person I love was being reduced to nothing.

Well, it's over for a while, and I'm going to try and prepare myself before the next meeting.

I wash my face in the lady's room and go to see Cal. He is dressed and cheerful, sitting in the dining room.

(155)

June 1999

June 6th

Today, Sunday, when I go down after church, Cal says, "You look so nice." I have on a suit and heels instead of the usual stuff. This is the first compliment Cal has given me in a long time. I love that he still notices what I wear.

June 25th

Our thirtieth anniversary. Thirty years. Where have they gone? How did we end up like this?

Outside rain drizzles down and the sky is a sullen gray. An overwhelming sadness settles around me. Thirty years ago, when Cal was forty-nine and I had just turned forty-three, anything and everything seemed possible. We were in love; we were married. We'd gotten a late start, but now that we'd begun, nothing could stop us, we thought. We were together, and that was all that mattered.

I remember our lawyer joking when we went to see him about our wills. "Cal, of course, doesn't need a will," he said. "He's going to outlive us all." It certainly seemed so. Both his mother and his father lived into their nineties. Cal didn't smoke, drank only an occasional Ballantine ale, and both his body and mind were in tip-top condition. We hadn't even heard the word *Alzheimer's*. And now where were we?

I look around the apartment at the furniture we brought from our old house——the white couch with its green and blue pillows and the drop-leaf table in front of the window, its sides almost touching the floor, that once belonged to my grandmother, as had the cherry chest with rough glass knobs, the caned chairs, the side tables. My mother's Audubon prints, the old painting Cal's parents brought back from Ireland.

It is attractive. It is all right. But what has happened to our plan to live together in our lovely house until we were very old? We'd roll around in our wheelchairs, we thought, with someone up in my office space who would cook and take care of us and not mind that we were still in love.

Tears stand in my eyes. I hate, hate Alzheimer's, that black, slimy serpent that slithered into our lives and smothered our joy.

The clock says ten in the morning. This is the time I go to be with Cal. But not today. I can't go today.

But by afternoon the rain has stopped. The skies are clearing, although some clouds still hang low. I miss Cal. I scold myself. Who are you to feel sorry for yourself when you've had a long, deep love affair of thirty years and more?

I take a shower, wash my hair, put on my blue linen suit, and go down to see Cal.

He is sitting in a chair in the space that serves as Whittier's living room. I stand in front of him. "Guess what, Cal? Today is our anniversary. We've been married thirty years."

Cal jumps out of his chair—the fastest I've seen him move in ages—wraps his arms around me, and says, "That's the best news I've heard in a long time."

I laugh out loud. Where did he find those words? "All right! Let's go celebrate."

I don't know exactly what Cal thinks is happening, but he is very happy, which is all I care about. We drive to a nearby café, find a table for two, and order a double scoop of vanilla ice cream with chocolate sauce, Cal's favorite, and two spoons. I raise a spoonful of ice cream and toast, "To many more."

Cal reaches across the table and taps his spoon against mine.

Somehow, regardless of the pain, as long as we're together, there are always scraps of joy.

July 1999

July 4th

Today is sunny and so is Cal. He is lying on his bed when I arrive. "Guess what?" I say. "We're going to a barbecue. I'm going to eat lunch with you."

"Great. Let's go."

And Cal is up and on his feet.

As we walk to the door, I ask, "Would you like to go to the bathroom?"

Usually, mention of the bathroom creates trauma, but not today. Cal answers affirmatively, he finishes in a couple of minutes, and we're back on track for the barbecue, which is located just outside of Whittier—a large flat grassy spot where picnic tables, benches, and an overflowing buffet have been set up.

We sit with some of our group from Whittier—Howard, Jane, Phyllis, Willie, and our nurses' aides, Kathy and Ginnie. I fill Cal's plate with potato salad, tomatoes, potato chips, and lemonade and cut up a hotdog for him. He finishes the first plate. I fix another. He finishes that too and tops it off with a bowl of cut-up cantaloupe.

Ginnie says, "Cal must've been a joy to cook for. Was there anything he didn't eat?"

"Not really," I say, thinking back to those long candlelit dinners as we told each other about our day and then how gradually, during the advance of Alzheimer's, our conversations slowed and petered out. Finally, before our move to Kendal, we were watching the news while we ate.

Those must have been frightening days for Cal. He fought so hard against the disease, at first by pretending nothing was wrong, later by volunteering for a research program, finally by refusing to cooperate, repeatedly fleeing the Friendship Program and asking, "Why do you want me to go down with the worst people?"

Now he has mostly given in. He rarely leaves the memory care unit, and I have to coax him out the door when we go for a ride. Whittier is what he knows, and he is reluctant to leave it.

July 14th

My son Steve has come all the way from Hawaii again, and it's so nice to have him here. He really wanted to spend some time with Cal as well as me and went down to Whittier yesterday. He said Cal willingly came out of his room to visit at a table in a corner of the living room and seemed to enjoy what Steve had to say, nodding, even smiling a bit. Then he put his head down on his arms, going to sleep or not wanting to listen any longer. Steve said he didn't mind; he felt they could spend time together in whatever way worked best for Cal, and just sat quietly with him at the table. After a bit Cal raised his head and gave Steve a small grin, and the two sat there a while longer, relaxing together.

This afternoon Steve went down to Whittier again and came back to say they had the same sort of visit, Steve talking a bit and then the two just sitting together at the table. Steve overheard one of the aides, apparently uncomfortable with the situation, ask the head nurse, Doris, whether she should do something, maybe take Cal back to his room.

"Oh no," Doris said. "That's Mary's son Steve. He's really good with Cal."

July 23rd

This morning I find Cal dressed, except again for his shoes, and smiling.

"Hi, Cal," I say. "I love you," and kiss him.

"Hi, Mary," he replies, smiling. "I love you too." Then for some reason today he asks, "Where do you live?"

"Right here in the same building as you. You have a room and I have a room in Kendal so I can come and see you lots each day."

Still smiling, Cal says, "That's nice."

I treasure these small pieces of happy conversation.

August 1999

Aug. 6th

Still, the stormy days grow more frequent.

"Shhh," says Cal as I arrive in Whittier. He is sitting in a chair in the dining room, and he motions with his arm to the other side of the room. I sit where he indicates and watch.

When the others in the room talk, Cal shouts, "Be quiet! Damn it! Be quiet!" and I know this will be one of the not-so-good days.

I turn to Cal. "Now," I say, "you need to be quiet too." And he is, although I have to repeat this a couple of times during the hour I'm there. I suggest a walk, a nap, some juice, a ride. They're all received with the same reply: "Shhh!"

Aug. 18th

Cal's decline continues. I attend another "progress" meeting. Again, each staff member reports on his or her latest interactions with Cal. "No longer able to put on socks." "No longer able to interact with staff members." "No longer able to whistle." On and on. Each statement makes me feel I am losing another part of Cal, when I am trying to hold on to and treasure what is left.

Mary MacCracken

I can't bear it. Why can't they say, "Still able to feed himself" or "Still able to walk slowly"? I ask if it is really necessary for me to be at the meetings, and they, the doctors and nurses, excuse me.

Aug. 21st

When I go down in the afternoon, Cal is lying on his bed but gets up willingly when I come in. When I ask if he'd like to go for a ride, he says, "Yes."

We drive down to a pretty pond nearby. On the way back we buy lemonade from two children sitting at a roadside stand they've set up. I can remember my excitement as a little girl when people actually bought what I had made.

I need gas and ask Cal if he'd mind if I stop to get it. I try to remember to treat Cal with the same courtesy as before he became ill, and he usually responds. He sits patiently while I pump and pay. I find myself constantly questioning, without words, the quality of Cal's life. It seems to vary, which I guess is fairly typical of the disease. Cal's doctors and some of the nurses have talked to me about whether I would want them to withhold antibiotics if Cal got pneumonia. No, I've always said. Now I'm not so sure.

September 1999

Sept. 6th

I had dinner last night with three women. One lost her husband from Parkinson's disease about a year ago. She seems strong and happy, planning her younger daughter's wedding in November. The old cliché about life moving on appears to be true.

I had planned to take Cal for a ride in the afternoon, but he is dozing in a chair in the dining room, shoes off, shirt and warm-up jacket off, not wanting to go anywhere. So I sit beside him and read the newspaper out loud to him as he dozes. Without a jacket or button-down shirt, his undershirt outlines his new small bulge of a stomach. Somehow it seems very endearing.

Sept. 14th

I take Cal to the music room. He mostly sits beside me with his eyes closed. I lean close to him and whisper, "Are you sleeping or hiding?"

He whispers back, "Both."

Mary MacCracken

Sept. 20th

Cal's son Mark was here this weekend. Cal was fine most of the time. He smiled several times, but when we tried to get him to hit a tennis ball with a racket, he didn't want to.

"Nobody does that," he said, meaning, we thought, that you play tennis on a tennis court, not on a walk in a garden. I was glad to hear him say what he did, because to me it meant he understood what was and what was not appropriate.

The only time Cal got upset was noon on Sunday. Things got kind of chaotic, and Cal refused to eat his lunch. I took him back to his room, and when I returned at three thirty, he was happy. We went for a ride. Cal said, "This is very nice." Later, "You do this so well."

I said, "I like being married to you."

"Me too," he replied.

October 1999

Oct. 5th

When I go down to see Cal around eleven in the morning, Doris, the head nurse of the unit, is waiting for me.

"Cal has had a really rough morning," she says. "He got up, dressed, ate breakfast, and then got almost physically violent with the nurses' aides. I told them to take him back to his room and let him calm down," she continued. "I went to see him later. He'd gotten off his shoes and socks and yelled at me, saying, 'Take those things off your face,' and grabbed at my glasses. He also tried to grab my keys out of my pocket. I don't know what's going on with him."

I thank Doris and walk on down to Cal's room—past the shower room where someone is shouting and a nurse is calling that she needs a bit of help. The climate at Whittier is like that—sometimes calm, sometimes stormy.

I'm not sure what to expect in Cal's room. He's lying on his bed, his eyes closed, one foot sticking out from under the covers.

"Hello," I say.

Cal opens his eyes and smiles. "Hello."

"I heard you were grumpy," I say.

"When was I grumpy?" he asks.

I put on his shoes and socks, and he stands up. Doris comes in. "How are you, my friend?" she asks.

Cal smiles. "Well, at least I got a smile," Doris says, before she leaves.

Oct. 10th

I never know now what mood to expect—sunny, sorrowful, or even angry. On this afternoon's visit I find Cal sitting in a chair in the dining room with his eyes closed. He doesn't respond when I greet him. I say, "You don't look quite as happy as you did this morning."

"That's right," he says, and closes his eyes.

Oct. 15th

Down in Whittier Cal has hated getting on the scales. Something about not having contact with the floor is frightening to him. But in early summer, one nurse was able to coax him to step up and stay long enough to record his weight, one hundred sixty-five pounds, a five-pound gain. I have become very fond of those five extra pounds. Somehow, they reassure me and make it seem that Cal is going to be around for a while. Besides, it evens things out. We have always been, and now still are, forty pounds apart.

Oct. 21st

But nothing is ever sure. The phone rings in my apartment at six thirty in the morning. "Mary. This is Fred Wilson, Cal's doctor."

My heart turns to ice. "Yes" is all I can say.

"Cal has pneumonia. I need to know whether you want him to have antibiotics or not?"

So we have reached this moment. I'm numb, stunned. I can't speak.

"Mary, I need your answer."

"Yes," I say again, not processing anything.

Gently, the doctor says, "I can order them. It's also all right not to order them, as you and I have talked about. It's up to you."

I hesitate, uncertain. "I need time to think," I say.

It isn't until later that I fully realize he was asking me if I wanted to let Cal die from pneumonia. Earlier I think I would have said no; it didn't seem like it was time.

I go down to Cal's room. A nurse is sitting beside Cal's bed. His eyes are closed. He's on oxygen. Plastic tubes are inserted in his nose. A machine is making a gurgling sound, or maybe it's Cal—I can't tell.

I turn to the nurse and say, "I'm here. It's okay if you go."

"No, ma'am. I'm on duty."

I can't imagine sitting in that room, with the nurse, listening to the machine or Cal breathe.

"I'll be back," I say and leave.

In our apartment, I put on my purple down jacket that Cal gave me, knitted wool cap, and gloves. It will be cold outside.

I need to think, which means I need to walk. I know nothing about pneumonia.

Oh, Cal, help me, I say to myself. *What would you want? I know what I want. I only want to keep you with me as long as possible.*

A voice speaks in my head. *It's obvious what you want, Mary. But how about Cal? What would he want?*

I try to turn the voice off, but it clearly says, *Do you think Cal likes living like this?*

I wipe my eyes before the tears can freeze.

"Of course not," I say out loud.

I go back to our apartment and call Cal's room.

"Yes?" says the nurse.

"This is Cal's wife. How is he?"

"No change."

I hang up and call Dr. Wilson.

"I've decided no antibiotics," I say.

"All right," he replies. "Is there anyone you want me to call?"

"Call?" I repeat.

"Yes. Family?"

Thinking of our combined seven children and their spouses and grandchildren, I say, "We have a lot of family."

"You can handle it?" he asks kindly.

"Yes, I think so."

I go back down to Cal's room in the afternoon. "No change," the nurse says.

I call in the evening. "No change," she says again.

Oct. 22nd

I call early in the morning. The phone in Cal's room rings on and on. *Oh, dear God* is my only thought.

I dial the nurses' station and ask, "Where's Cal? No one answered when I called his room."

"That's because he's just down the hall eating his breakfast."

"Breakfast? He wasn't able to breathe by himself last night."

"Well, he's much better now. Never can tell about pneumonia. Different every time."

Cal is not only better. He is much, much better. When I next see Cal, he's up, he is shaved, he is dressed. His eyes are bright; he's smiling. He doesn't tilt his face up to be kissed. Instead, he reaches out and hugs me to him, saying, "There you are. I've been waiting for you."

"Well, here I am. You look wonderful. Are they giving you some new medicine?"

"Nope. No medicine at all. No pill. No potions. No paregoric. Only good food."

Oh, maybe that's it, I think. *Maybe this is how he is when he's not all doped up.* It's been so long since Cal joked around that I've forgotten how to reply.

Oct. 25th

Cal smiles when he recognizes me. He sits in a straight chair with the others until it is time for lunch. The group is doing nursery rhymes with the new music therapist. She or an aide gives clues, and the residents fill in the missing words. Except for Cal. He sits with closed eyes, smiling occasionally. This morning the day care children have been in to make paper skunks. I say that Cal and his friends once brought home baby skunks when he was eight. One girl asks Cal if this is true. He answers with his eyes still closed, nodding. "Yes, it is," he says.

For lunch there is macaroni and cheese, beets, potato puffs, and milk and some dessert. When I begin pouring Margaret's milk, Cal says, "Where's mine? I don't have any." He takes up his fork and eats eagerly.

But our blessed time of reprieve is soon over.

November 1999

Nov. 4th

Cal is ill again and has been all week. They said at first it was an upper respiratory inflammation, but it doesn't sound very upper to me now. He has a deep cough with phlegm, and a fever of 101 degrees.

The unit is quiet and somewhat sad. Several others are sick, and Willie has fallen again, banging his head. Cal is in bed, asleep. He wakes and looks at me without expression and then recognizes me. His face lights up. He speaks a little, the first half-dozen words making sense and then trailing off. I try to tie my responses into what I think he is trying to say.

Nov. 5th

The trees in Hanover swirl in the wind and flaunt their colors, but there is also a sense of something ending. I feel it in my bones.

Cal isn't eating; his round stomach has disappeared. Even though I still mash, butter, and cut his food, he doesn't want to eat.

"Maybe," I say to the head nurse, "his throat hurts or his stomach. Maybe we should ask one of his doctors to take a look."

"Maybe," she replies, "Cal knows something we don't."

I begin to ache, not in any particular place but all over.

Nov. 6th

Cal's favorite nurse, Ellen, stops me this morning as I enter Whittier. Somewhat shaken, she says that Cal just told her: "I'm going to die soon. But I want to thank you all for taking good care of me."

She pauses. "I thought you should know, Mary."

I shake my head. Cal is only seventy-nine; his parents lived into their nineties. *Cal,* I think silently, *you can do that too. If your parents did, you can too.* I don't say it out loud, but I think it. Now I realize this is what they call denial.

But I do stop pushing dinners of meat and potatoes or chicken and rice and instead ask the kitchen for dishes of orange ice. I don't know why; it just seems right, and Cal swallows each spoonful eagerly.

Nov. 9th

Cal sleeps now, through the days, through the nights. He has pneumonia again and is put on oxygen once more. The nurse tells me it makes it easier for him, and brings in a chair so I can sit close to his bed, but I need more. I need body contact. I need to be able to touch him, but his arms and hands are tightly tucked beneath the sheets, I suppose so he won't disturb his oxygen tubes. I settle for his ankle. Cal only turns and looks at me once. All he says is "There you are."

I know what he means. I answer, "Always."

I sit beside him into the night. He wakes again. He says my

name and then "I love you." He couldn't have given me a better gift.

Nov. 10th

I sit beside Cal for sixteen hours, from early morning on. His daughter Joan, a doctor, arrives at ten at night. I rise to greet her, and we talk for a minute or two, but then she puts her finger to her lips and says, "He's gone."

I put my face against his and it's true; he isn't there. Pneumonia has given him the exit he deserved. One of the two nurses who sit across the room says, "You can say goodbye now."

I feel an unreasonable jolt of anger. I want to say, "Please get out. Just go." I want, need, a moment of privacy to say, "Cal, please take me with you."

But I say nothing. I just kiss him and then only whisper, "Thank you," hoping he can somehow hear me thank him for so many things . . .

Not for the beginning this time, Cal, but for the end. Thank you for your courage in being open about your illness, saying outright almost as soon as you knew, "I have a little bit of Alzheimer's." Thank you for always believing you could win against the disease, fighting it as you fought back on tennis and squash courts. You almost had me believing too. "We'll beat Alzheimer's," you said, "and then we'll write a book about it." Of course, we didn't. But it didn't beat us either. We stayed close and loving in spite of it, and our last years together were still sweet.

If you can, Cal, stay close to me now. Help me be stronger, braver than I know how to be by myself. Help me to go out and go on, with grace. I will always love you. Thank you.

Epilogue

Christmas Day 2000

Today at dawn, I'm still dreaming. I often have dreams, but I don't usually remember them. However, there is one I will never forget—and maybe, maybe it wasn't a dream.

About a month ago, a year after Cal died, I hear a voice in the middle of the night saying, "Hello, darling."

I can't see anyone, but I know the voice—"Cal, is that you?"

"It is indeed."

"How did you get down here?" I ask.

"Well, I invented a little jet engine that I wear right between my shoulder blades, and I can fly most any place."

"Oh," I say, "does everybody up there wear those now?"

"No," he answers, "the women still like their wings. Anyway, the reason I'm here is to tell you something important. I know you've always believed that after you die, you'll return to earth in some form or other. You claim God wouldn't be wasteful, but I want you to know it doesn't work that way. Once you're up here, you're up here for good. So, anything you want to do on earth you've got to get done now."

I know what he means: the book we were going to write about Alzheimer's. I don't want to talk about that now. I want to hear more about him.

"Okay. But how are you? How long can you stay?"

"Actually, my time is up. I picked up a bunch of demer-its while I was trying out my shoulder jet engine. A few little crashes, things like that, you know."

"Will you be back?"

"Yes, they say the longer you're up there, the more time you get down here. Being invisible, though, you can't do very much. You know I love you and always will."

There was never a face, and now the voice is gone. But still, I wake up smiling.

It has never happened again, but I figure he's probably work-ing on a new invention, and there are always a few "crashes" during an invention. One of these days I'll hear that voice again.

In the meantime, I'll be working on our book.

Acknowledgments

This book took a very long time to write, in part as my mother, Mary MacCracken, first had to recover from losing Cal. Friends at Kendal helped, especially Betsy and Sandy Sanderson, Margo Johnson, and Carol Mae Encherman, as did meetings both before and after Cal's death with Ruth Whybrow, the social worker whose skillful approach my mother describes in the book.

A key role was played by Mary Otto, who led the writing group that enabled my mother to start this book and then carry on with it. Her enthusiastic support of my mother's writing and her excellent editorial suggestions, especially as to how to pull all the bits and pieces into a reasonable order, were invaluable. Thanks also to everyone in the writing group, for their comments and support, and Mary Jenkins in particular, in part for driving my mother to the meetings in her last years. Gene Young, whose astute editorial advice helped shape my mother's first books, once again provided encouragement and suggestions for improvements. Thanks to those at She Writes Press, especially Samantha Strom, and to publicist Caitlin Hamilton Summie, for all their hard work. Thanks also to my mother's cousin, Nancy Seeley, for, among many other things, printing out an early draft of the book at the St. Lawrence River;

to Meredith Kurose, Joan Linsenmeier, Linda MacCracken, Karen McCahill, and Janine McKee for reading the manuscript in its last stages and making useful corrections; and to my brother Steve Thistle for supporting its publication.

In terms of dealing with Alzheimer's itself, the whole family, especially Cal's four children, provided an immense, unflagging and essential amount of help, far beyond that detailed in the book. Thanks also to so many others mentioned in its pages, among them Nancy Dubler for her kind advice in the early stretch of Alzheimer's and to Dr. Robert Santulli, for his wise and gentle care of Cal, and my mother as well. Anyone facing Alzheimer's needs a doctor like him. He also provided useful feedback on the book and a great foreword. As is clear in the book, Kendal at Hanover was a major source of support for my mother and Cal. Heartfelt thanks to Kendal and its workers. We need more retirement communities like this.

My mother died before this book was published. Writing it was a major part of almost every day until the end of her life. She always reread her latest draft (her first, and second, and third, and so on), penciling in corrections and improvements. She also took many copies of this or that chapter to her writing group, carefully collecting all these at the end of each meeting and bringing them home to go over the comments made in their margins. This resulted in a massive amount, pages and pages, of material and many revisions to incorporate suggestions. A major task was getting a clear, clean draft of the book in one place, in one computer file, and printed out and placed in one big red three-ring notebook, with all the other pages taken to the recycle bin. Whew! This was no easy job. Then my mother sat with this notebook, and the several that followed as each new draft was printed out, reading through

Mary MacCracken

the pages, making further corrections and edits, improving the manuscript more and more. She made it the very best she could. Thanks to her for writing this book. Thanks again also to all who helped her get it written, including her husband Cal MacCracken.

Susan L. Thistle

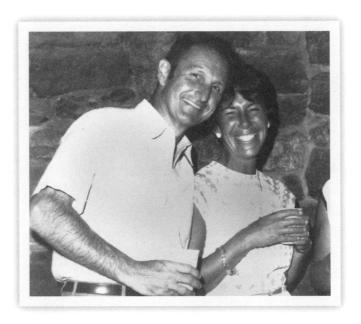

Cal and Mary MacCracken
Fridstol, Yelping Hill
Early Days

About the Author

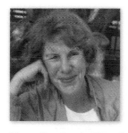

Mary MacCracken, an internationally best-selling author, wrote four earlier books about her work with autistic and learning-disabled children: *Circle of Children* (republished as *Lost Children*), *Lovey, City Kid,* and *Turn-About Children* (republished as *A Safe Place for Joey*). Her books have been published in fourteen countries and the first two were made into movies for television, starring the actress Jane Alexander. Mary spent her last years with her husband, Cal, an inventor with eighty patents, at Kendal at Hanover, a Continuous Care Retirement Community in Hanover, New Hampshire, and the decade after his death writing about their experiences dealing with his disease.

SELECTED TITLES FROM SHE WRITES PRESS

She Writes Press is an independent publishing
company founded to serve women writers everywhere.
Visit us at www.shewritespress.com.

Her Beautiful Brain: A Memoir by Ann Hedreen. $16.95, 978-1-938314-92-6. The heartbreaking story of a daughter's experiences as her beautiful, brainy mother begins to lose her mind to an unforgiving disease: Alzheimer's.

Don't Leave Yet: How My Mother's Alzheimer's Opened My Heart by Constance Hanstedt. $16.95, 978-1-63152-952-8. The chronicle of Hanstedt's journey toward independence, self-assurance, and connectedness as she cares for her mother, who is rapidly losing her own identity to the early stage of Alzheimer's.

Searching for Normal: The Story of a Girl Gone Too Soon by Karen Meadows. $16.95, 978-1-63152-137-9. Karen Meadows intertwines her own story with excerpts from her daughter Sadie's journals to describes their roller coaster ride through Sadie's depression and a maze of inadequate mental health treatment and services—one that ended with Sadie's suicide at age eighteen.

Flip-Flops After Fifty: And Other Thoughts on Aging I Remembered to Write Down by Cindy Eastman. $16.95, 978-1-938314-68-1. A collection of frank and funny essays about turning fifty—and all the emotional ups and downs that come with it.

Role Reversal: How to Take Care of Yourself and Your Aging Parents by Iris Waichler. $16.95, 978-1-63152-091-4. A comprehensive guide for the 45 million people currently taking care of family members who need assistance because of health-related problems.

The Shelf Life of Ashes: A Memoir by Hollis Giammatteo. $16.95, 978-1-63152-047-1. Confronted by an importuning mother 3,000 miles away who thinks her end is nigh—and feeling ambushed by her impending middle age—Giammatteo determines to find The Map of Aging Well, a decision that leads her on an often-comic journey.

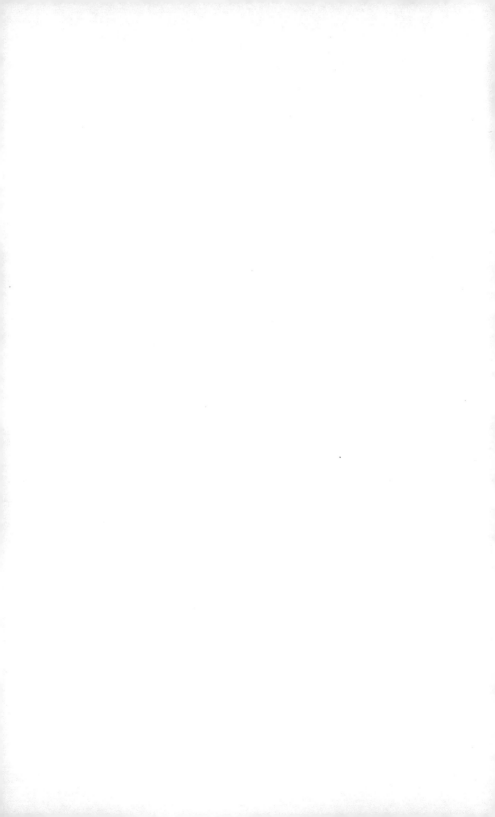